Research in the development of effective services for hearing-impaired people

FIFTH
H.M. QUEEN ELIZABETH
THE QUEEN MOTHER FELLOWSHIP

1993

Research in the development of effective services for hearing-impaired people

PROFESSOR MARK HAGGARD

Medical Research Council
Institute of Hearing Research
Nottingham

THE NUFFIELD PROVINCIAL
HOSPITALS TRUST

Published by the
Nuffield Provincial Hospitals Trust
3 Prince Albert Road, London NW1 7SP

ISBN 0 900574 82 8

Designed by Bernard Crossland

PRINTED IN GREAT BRITAIN BY
BURGESS (ABINGDON) LTD
THAMES VIEW, ABINGDON
OXFORDSHIRE

HER MAJESTY QUEEN ELIZABETH THE QUEEN MOTHER FELLOWSHIP

Her Majesty Queen Elizabeth the Queen Mother,
who is the Patron of the Trust and has
always shown a keen interest in its work,
approved the founding of the Fellowship
by the Trust to commemorate her
80th birthday.

The Trustees of the Nuffield Provincial
Hospitals Trust will select a Fellow who
will be invited to undertake to review
in a monograph a subject within the
sphere of the Trust which is believed to
be of particular interest to Her Majesty.
The monograph will be launched by
a lecture

CONTENTS

PREFACE

IN THIS MONOGRAPH I WRITE AS AN APPLIED SCIENTIST CLOSELY
allied to medicine. Medical scientists seek to provide applicable
generalisations and techniques for doctors and non-medical professionals, as well as for decision-makers in health care, and they
ultimately serve the public through the cumulative actions of all
these groups. The term 'applied' suggests hopes of seeing research
disseminated into application, and some obligation to expedite
that process. Many issues arise about how decisions to implement
are to be taken and how implementation is to be encouraged.
Many scientists regard implementation as the responsibility of
others for understandable reasons. The 'downstream' stages between basic research and application can be expensive or
frustrating, and they are not always the best use of researchers'
time and particular skills. Promising findings can eventually be
rendered inapplicable in several ways: through being over-taken
by more radical developments, or through a change, disappear-
ance or a failure to develop the appropriate professional
responsibilities and skills. Because of this application gap, the
scientist content to leave the steps towards implementation totally
to someone else may end up doing inapplicable science, or science
that is, or was, applicable but never actually applied. Results are
unlikely to be applied unless they have been anticipated with an
application stage in view and make use of the concept of cost
alongside that of benefit. The mechanisms for research to underpin health care have been imperfect in the past, and there has
been increasing determination recently to overcome the
deficiencies in the mechanisms for having research implemented.[1]
Some stake or obligation on the part of the researcher in the
eventual application of new principles is obviously one way to
make research relevant. If research has answered the right questions, failures to achieve application in the health sphere most

References begin on p. xiv.

ix

commonly arise through institutional obstacles to implementation, in which shortage of resources plays a contributory but not
always an overriding role. Application often faces difficulties in
realising the savings on dismantling what is old in order to invest
in what is new. Investment decisions on implementation in the
health sphere are often forced but rarely made by research
scientists.

Implementation embraces professional, managerial and even
political issues in which scientists are often wary of becoming
entangled; some of these are touched on in Chapters 1 and 5. As
in scholastic debate, individual scientists have to decide just how
deeply to become involved in inter-professional or even political
debates on service provision; compromising their impartiality may
restrict their longer-term influence as providers of the impartial
data and interpretations that are needed in policy decisions. The
threats to impartiality are particularly high when a scientist or
research-oriented clinician is involved in all stages: the proposal of
a new development, its evaluation, and the decision to implement—precisely that longitudinal span and involvement that is
desirable for other reasons, such as to aid implementation. In
some instances tension between the roles appropriate to each
stage may be of little consequence, but where resource implications are high the stages should be separated in the interests of
impartiality.

Many scientists avoid publicity and public debate. There is a
tendency among politicians, on their experience of a few scientists
with high profiles, to write off all scientists as just another professional lobby or interest group—a mistake that society as a whole
can ill afford. One aspect of scientific involvement therefore
requires a special comment, the separation of scientific findings,
particularly those which underpin public health policy, from the
advocacy undertaken by voluntary associations and pressure
groups. As an example of this dilemma, for me to wave the banner
for hearing-impaired people in a partisan way might make a good
read for some, but it would lead to a loss of objectivity and could
alienate others from important messages in the data which I
report; this would not ultimately help hearing-impaired people.
Voluntary organisations are a necessary part of that pluralistic
web of exchanges whereby society allocates the scale and nature
of appropriate provision for its members' various needs. In these

exchanges, dialogue is required between medical scientists and voluntary organisations, just as it is required with other stake-holders: with managers, with the professions, including public health specialists, and with government. However, the scientist should avoid becoming exclusively identified with the current stance adopted by any particular stake-holder. The priorities of these different groups, the relative magnitudes of health problems, and the preferred solutions are all evolving continuously in ways that complicate the scientist's job. Equally, scientific evidence evolves over time. Dialogue among the stake-holders may be sporadic, but it must be continuous, not once-and-for-all.

If I have any banner to wave, it is that of the systems theorist— one who believes that the human benefits from bio-medicine and related technologies can be large, but that realising them requires us also to understand the complex and variable human, techno-logical and socio-economic systems that deliver those benefits. In the present context this requires a systematic understanding of the health care system. Such understanding underpins successful implementation. It requires the analysis and evaluation of profes-sional procedures and health care delivery systems, using scientific concepts of measurement, control and statistical inference, as well as an understanding of the primary phenomena of disease and treatment. Such analysis is the way to arrive at firm recommenda-tions on what could and should be done, and on how best to do it; hence I conclude this monograph with a short section on health service research (HSR) within Chapter 5.

In order to emphasise the public health aspects of hearing problems, I have had to omit discussion of many aspects of hear-ing impairment, both scientific and vocational. For example, much of the professional care given to profoundly deaf people falls outside the health sphere; for the signing members of the deaf community this care falls in particular to social workers and for pre-lingually hearing-impaired children to teachers of the deaf. I respect both the case work undertaken by these professions and their wishes for the firmer scientific underpinning that a sustained research effort would bring. I regret that I can offer these pro-fessions outside the health sector only some epidemiological background information, as the requirements of the health sector have been large enough to preoccupy me.

Where multiple perspectives and several professions are concerned with one problem area, there is always the potential danger of confusion and non-communication through the adoption of conflicting or diverging terminologies. A nice example is the term 'common', which to social workers means 'shared' and hence has a high value attached to it, but to most clients of social workers means 'cheap and nasty'. In audiology 'benefit' is a measure of health gain rooted in auditory performance, for example the advantages to communication conferred by using a hearing aid; it is not a social security entitlement or transfer payment. Additionally, in economics a cost-benefit analysis assumes that benefits can be reduced to financial terms, whereas a cost-utility analysis does not. 'Benefit' in audiology therefore equates more to the economist's 'utility'. Thus the reader will have to tolerate some local usages and discussion of how certain terms and definitions have arisen. Even where I do not advocate replacing the term in question, reflection upon usage is usually justified as revealing underlying conflicts in conceptualisation on possibilities of misunderstanding. Some of my own terminology may jar, for example the use of the now widespread word 'professionals' to describe both the doctors and non-doctors in a particular field. The reader may feel that some such usages are unnecessary jargon, but the 1000 words of basic English were not chosen for describing complex socio-technical systems in unambiguous ways.

My two main chapters discuss hearing impairment in middle and old age, and the early detection of hearing impairment in children, including otitis media. The particular problems chosen are heavily biased towards issues that research by my colleagues and myself has addressed; the citations are biased in the same way. This monograph is intended not as a comprehensive academic review but as an illustration of how a field can be advanced by the work of a research institute in it. Aspects of the material used have in most instances been, or are being, published in peer-reviewed journals. The Nuffield Provincial Hospitals Trust invites its Fellows to re-cross old ground in a new direction. The attraction and advantage of this for the writer and for the professional reader lie in the comparison and reflection upon aspects of applied knowledge, especially those with implications for service delivery, that may have had to be relegated to brief asides or scattered footnotes in primary publications to avoid editorial expurgation.

One of my aims has been to produce a monograph which

insiders (in this case audiologists, otolaryngologists and other specialists) will find useful alongside primary sources, and which incorporates concepts not previously or widely seen within these disciplines, so encouraging them to look outwards to health services research and public health issues. My second aim is that outsiders (for example, managers, public health professionals, and epidemiologists) should find the specialist material presented in an accessible way that kindles a general interest in hearing and in applications with the hearing-impaired, while also introducing the high level of scientific sophistication now being achieved. Audiologists and otologists have presented neither the problems they tackle nor their successes sufficiently to the wider audience, and the barrier of a technical vocabulary is in part to blame. I have been directly involved in both the areas of research chosen, so have attempted to explain and justify some of the intellectual threads that drive the research in the two problem areas. In my experience, generalists are more likely to foster the maintenance, extension and application of knowledge about hearing and hearing impairment once they know something about it. There should be some advantages to them in a presentation wherein the technical aspects are summarised beyond some basic audiological facts necessary to formulate the service problems. As an aim for a short monograph to spread this understanding widely is a long shot. If I do not fully succeed here, I hope at least to convince the reader that the enterprise is worthwhile and worth following to completion in other publications.

Much of my material serves to convey a sense of how health services do and should evolve, rather than concentrating on precise current details, which are likely to change greatly. I know from previous experiences that some readers will describe this monograph as 'speculative'—now a term undeservedly used in a derogatory way for the absence of an exclusive preoccupation with minor modifications to facts already established. Because it is necessarily concerned with chains of argument, I prefer to describe the approach as 'propositional'. I regard this quality as necessary where decisions to change health services are faced that will entrain large resources and large potential differences in human health and well-being. Without propositions to debate or evaluate, scientists, doctors, managers and politicians cannot communicate, cannot envisage possible futures and cannot make wise

PREFACE

decisions. Unfortunately the truth and relevance of some of the crucial propositions are uncertain, through lack of the relevant facts. I have felt it proper not to conceal such uncertainties from purchasers or providers of health care, but I do not throw up my hands either. To arrive at the greater eventual certainties which the design of appropriate services requires also requires propositions. Thus, my third aim is to boost the critical discussion of **rationale**, which I found in the recent review of the screening of children's hearing[2] to be so deficient, at the centre of discussions of research and services. Unfortunately the pressures for brevity in medical publication favour minor variations on the conventional, at the expense of rationale and of conceptual clarification. The invitation by the Nuffield Provincial Hospitals Trust to produce this monograph is therefore most welcome.

REFERENCES

1. RICHARDSON, A., JACKSON, C., AND SYKES, W., (1990). *Taking Research Seriously: Means of improving and assessing the use and dissemination of research.* HMSO, London.
2. HAGGARD, M. P., AND HUGHES, E., (1991). *Screening Children's Hearing: A review of the literature and the implications of Otitis Media.* HMSO, London.

LIST OF FIGURES

LIST OF TABLES

1

SPECIAL PROBLEMS IN DEVELOPING EFFECTIVE SERVICES FOR THE DISABILITIES: THE WIDER CONTEXT OF RESEARCH

IN HEALTH CARE, AND FOR THE DISABILITIES IN PARTICULAR, THE obstacles and difficulties to improving services are many. Research can contribute both at the level of changing attitudes to need and possibilities (policy research) and at the detailed levels of practical solutions and their evaluation. To realise this potential, an understanding of the origins and nature of these obstacles is necessary. The feasible time course of improvements to the human condition usually turns out to be longer than hoped by researchers or the professionals applying research. This chapter addressed eight issues specific to the disabilities and two others general to applied research. The reader already widely experienced in research in health or disabilities and its application may wish to sample the italicised conclusions of each section and perhaps read only sections 4, 6 and 8.

In clinical medicine, anecdotes are nowadays deplored as a basis for practice, being rightly replaced by knowledge of a more systematically acquired type, including that gained by clinical trials. However a good story has didactic value, and my first two points are most succinctly illustrated by true stories. Both happened in North European countries outside the UK, with comparable high standards of scientific achievement and state welfare provision. One I experienced myself; one was told to me by a scientist who was personally involved.

References begin on p. 30.

1. GENERALISTS AND SPECIALISTS

In country A, the department of local government was drawing up a specification for sheltered housing for the elderly. The planner thought that resources could 'reasonably' be spared and more effectively deployed, by lowering the usual standards for acoustic isolation in and between the dwelling units. His stereotype assumed that the residents, tending to have at least mild hearing impairments, would be less bothered by sound penetration than the average citizen. Consultation spread as far as a research scientist who studies hearing. He pointed out the fallacy in the planner's assumption that the only concern should be annoyance from attenuated sound passing between the dwelling units. Rather, **higher** standards of acoustic isolation were actually required (and were duly adopted) for two reasons: (a) some hearing-impaired people turn the volume on their radios and televisions up very high, hence special provision may be necessary for the amenity of others; (b) the forms of hearing impairment that are closely allied to ageing involve an inability to distinguish wanted from unwanted sounds; sounds much above the threshold of hearing do not appear any less loud than they do to normally-hearing people. In psycho-acoustic jargon this is called loss of selectivity; it leads in effect to a loss of signal-to-noise ratio in the auditory nervous system. This inability entails a need to **keep out** noise from adjacent buildings and to **dampen out** internal reverberations (which have an effect similar to that of unwanted noise). To be fair to the planners of country A, this realisation had only spread from physiologists and psycho-acousticians to audiologists around 1980 and is only now beginning to spread among other relevant professions.

The sheltered housing story illustrates two points. Firstly, policy in general aspects of welfare provision such as housing cannot proceed in the language of administration and the social sciences alone. Technical understanding from fundamental research has to feed directly into policy and policy change, as well as being filtered into recurrent practice in professional disciplines. Secondly, stereotypes and suppositions about people that seem to stem from 'common sense' can be downright inaccurate, and this is as true in the area of hearing impairment as in any other.

Uncompromising specialists are required to understand normal sensory processes and pathology, and to develop effective technologies or regimes of care, dispelling old fallacies as they progress. A separate and complementary perspective (generalist, or at least embracing several further disciplines) is also required to consider questions of priority, the gain to public health, difficulties in implementation and the implications for training, job-descriptions and recruitment of the professionals that deliver health care. Some individuals can embrace both these perspectives, but the benefits of combination are most widely and reliably assured by partnerships of individuals with differing backgrounds—multidisciplinarity. To underline the importance of the partnership between specialist and generalist I continue in this chapter to interleave discussion of types of problem that are widespread in the delivery of health care with specialised facts and principles about hearing and hearing disorders.

Conclusion: Specialists and generalists need each other; generalists who do not know much about hearing can make serious mistakes.

2. INFLUENCE AND CONFLICT

My second anecdote concerns an international conference on technology for the disabled. In the host country B the statutory body representing the consumer (i.e. disabled people) had threatened to withdraw its support from the conference. This occurred because the chosen auditorium, complete with public address and induction loop system, had been built before the 1970s and was a stair-climb above the topmost floor accessible by the lift; hence there was no wheelchair access. The meeting had to be held in the basement, in a room with bleak lighting and abysmal reverberant acoustics. I saw no person with a wheelchair actually turn up to any of the meetings. However one major participant long blind and obviously unable to lip-read, was particularly reliant on his (deteriorating) hearing. The absence in the basement of an induction loop or even a public address system made the meeting frustrating and unproductive for him. To avoid embarrassing my host in B, I have refrained till now from making the two points illustrated by this imposed and counter-productive barter of wheelchair access for tolerable acoustics. Firstly, interests of groups within society—even within the disabled as a whole—

stand in some degree of conflict, often directly so. Secondly, the voicing of these interests, and the responses to them by administration, management or government are somewhat arbitrary processes; as in other political processes, ideology, tradition, individual charisma, stereotype · and *force majeure* may win over fairnesss, and even over pragmatism. The decisions that are taken may receive some scrutiny for precedent or even for cost, benefit and risk, but rarely for hidden opportunity costs.

I continue to draw a further lesson from this anecdote: claims to represent the consumer's interest can have a motherhood-and-apple-pie quality; they come stamped with the implication that they stand above disciplined analysis or questioning. One source of information about consumers' interests is indeed such direct political advocacy by their representatives. This is necessary but insufficient, and on its own can be unbalanced. Three other balancing sources of such information are: satisfaction surveys, the epidemiology of need, and the operation of forms of market (if these can be created or supported so as to function with high freedom and high quality of information, which is not always possible).

It is possible to view provision for the needs of any group of disabled people as essentially a political struggle for emancipation. The history of indifference, hostility and offensive representations as a burden within society makes excesses such as that in the previous anecdote very understandable. These conflicts have a parallel in research also, via the framework of assumptions upon which projects are chosen, and how they are formulated, interpreted and published. Three styles of research on disability can be distinguished which emerged in different periods but are all still current. They are, in historical sequence: (i) the positivist or objective (natural science) approach, seeking to describe and explain impairment, disability and handicap as properties of the individual; (ii) the interpretative (social science) approach, in which disability is seen as a societal problem; (iii) the emancipatory approach in which the context is an essentially political struggle. It would be biased and naive to reject the sociological analysis of the process of research production that leads to these distinctions or to deny that in the past research has been performed upon the weak by the powerful, but almost never in the reverse relationship. Once the research worker has thought through the implications of these styles of analysis there is a form of conversion of philosophy[1] from which returning is difficult if not impossible. This so-called 'action research' may serve the valuable function of freeing disabled people from unnecessary and inappropriate feelings of rejection, guilt and inadequacy. What is less clear is whether it can lead to cumulative and applicable knowledge when it emerges from a struggle for emancipation or is even properly called 'research'. The facts it establishes include facts about people's subjective worlds, which are sought in a selective and active way, to buttress the steps in a political argument not merely limited by cultural blinkers. Interpretative research has been seen as not succeeding in the delivery of tangible benefits even by critics of positivist research.[2] With these cross-currents, there is great potential for disability research to be contentious or even confused. The perspective that positivist research confers is at best restricted because it does not claim that people's feelings fall within its scope. It does not necessarily contribute to the climate whereby society or individuals decided to take action to remedy matters and it can occasionally at its worst be dehumanising. How can a positivist researcher such as myself admit such propositions yet carry on doing positivist research?

The concept of cultural inevitability comes to the rescue here. The objective, positivist paradigm tends to be useful for providing data that will improve rehabilitative engineering and documenting the types of need that might be met 'from the outside', for example by changes in transfer payments, in service delivery mechanisms or in other things that result from structured action using resources of which society as a whole disposes. Positivist research remains that style of research that carries most guarantees of usefulness. Whether and how it becomes used is an important question, but not a research question. These are the axioms of the research culture into which I was socialised, and a sufficiently convincing case has not yet been made for advantages accruing to anyone if I were to abandon these axioms, provided that my positivist research is guided and informed by the above admissions.

Conclusion: It is best to proceed by priorities and targets for improving conditions for each disabled group in a pragmatic fashion. Overdependence on ideological principles, advocacy and rights, or on piecemeal legislation, can lead to chaos. Any vacuum will be filled by the views of the most vocal or most powerful group. This principle includes the dominance in welfare provision and in research formulation by people who are not themselves disabled, but the practical advantages that would flow from radical change are not evident.

3. WHAT MATTERS MOST?

Doctors and scientists who work on cancer treatment have until recently said that lives—survival rates or survival times—matter most, and that the application of quality-of-life measures is at best premature. Their main concern is developing therapeutic regimes that influence survival at all, or by (say) 10 per cent more than previous regimes, so this concentration on mortality is a useful way for researchers to focus immediately on a clear-cut indicator of efficacy where the ultimate aim of eliminating a particular cancer as a cause of death remains far off. However, patients and their families sometimes tell a more subtle story that puts greater emphasis on the quality of life. The tension between concern for mortality on the one hand, and concern for the trio of morbidity, disability and distress on the other, has been addressed systematically in recent years. This is a particularly important tension for work in hearing impairment, which has negligible association with mortality but a very high prevalence and high impact on the quality of life.

It is now widely appreciated that containment of the killers of youth and middle age has led to new patterns of morbidity and disability in survivors. Are the steady improvements in life expectancy over the last two centuries quite as beneficial as they look, once this morbidity and disability are taken into account? At the margin, what balance of resources should now go into the further prolongation of life *versus* the improvement in its quality? The answer to the first question is rather complicated, due to the many assumptions that must be made when bringing sets of data into register with one another across sex, socio-economic group, time, or place and across type of disease or disability. The hope of entirely avoiding terminal morbidity and disability is, of course, not realistic. However it is not clear that there have been sufficient health gains for the survivors in the seventh and eighth decades of life truly to compress morbidity and disability into the last few years as hoped. Several sets of data suggest a static distribution of morbidity and disability over age, with more people surviving to be ill and disabled. Such a 'failure of success' would imply a consequently **increased proportion** of the average life affected by age related disability.[3] Data from England and Wales[4] do indeed suggest increases in the proportion of life with disability both for men and women, although there has been a small absolute increase in disability-free years for men. Whilst further analyses of this type on a wide range of health indicators are called for, examination so far suggests a slightly pessimistic conclusion: disease and disability have not yet been compressed into the final few years of the life-span.

The issue of morbidity compression invokes an apparent conflict between saving lives and enhancing lives. To raise the issue does not necessarily question the value of the achievements in life expectancy—for the individual the balance depends on the degree of disability and on other aspects of the quality of life permitted. However, for society the justification for spending further resources on saving lives becomes coupled to the prospects either of deferring morbidity and disability by preventive measures, or of greatly reducing the impact of these on the general quality of life by compensatory prosthetics, rehabilitation or adjustments and compensation in the social sphere. A clear implication emerges from this discussion that the duration of life free from disability and disease should now become the major gross performance indicator for health programmes, whether preventative or reactive. This is sometimes called HALE (healthy active life expectancy) or, less positively, quality-adjusted survival.

Reviews of morbidity and mortality data[3,4,5] have shown an interesting comparison between major causes of ill-health in respect of how they influence morbidity and disability *versus* mortality. As might be expected, circulatory disease, neoplastic disease (cancer) and accidents top the ranking for reducing life-expectancy. These would thus rank top for implementation of service improvements if radical innovations leading to improvements in life-expectancy were to come along. For **disability-free** life expectancy, circulatory disease enters again, now followed by locomotor disorders, respiratory disorders and sensory impairments. (Note that these are broad and potentially over-lapping categories, rather than cognate ones: cancer refers to a class of pathological process, whilst locomotor disorders refer to a domain of consequences of pathology in any of several different physiological systems. Nor are the disease groups independent; circulatory disorders also contribute to sensory disorders.) Robine and Ritchie's analysis[5] based on old US data places sensory disorders only fourth in the prevalence ranking but ahead of four other groups tabulated. More up-to-date data suggest higher prevalence for sensory disorders.* Of the many assumptions that the construction of such league tables must make, two of importance are the appropriateness and the scaling of the measures used, and the adoption of a particular cut-off for the degree of severity to include in the analysis.

Public health strategies have inevitably to make some questionable assumptions in the attempt to equate severities in different areas of functioning. It is often said by people who have lost their hearing and by their families, particularly if the deterioration in hearing was rapid, that the social isolation is worse than they could have imagined and that the isolation and mental distress are worse than mere pain. How could this contention be tested and calibrated? It would be impracticable to compose a sample of people suffering doubly from various pairs of disabilities and to ask them to compare the respective disabilities or handicap (or perhaps the subjective feelings about these) against objective measures of the impairment in question, and then to cross-calibrate modalities of disability in such a sample. A number of attempts have been made to achieve usable equivalences of verbal questionnaire responses. In a UK study of all the disabilities by OPCS,[6] a panel of judges comprising specialists from each area plus generalists rated a range of items for several areas of disability. This comparison and other comparisons of this type place

---

*Multi-modal disability surveys generally compute prevalences from verbal responses only. This can lead to problems: OPCS used a 'screen' pre-question to exclude levels of disability below some level thought to be worth documenting, before further counting and comparing the disabilities. A prevalence of only 5.9% was estimated for hearing impairment in the adult disability survey, as against the 25.6% for a nominally similar question in the National Study of Hearing. The consequent comparisons by OPCS between areas of disability may have grossly underestimated the prevalence for hearing impairments that are worthy of concern. Whether the cut-offs should generally be set at mild or severe levels overall is a separate issue.

being totally unable to hear on a par with being totally unable to see or to speak, but some way short of being totally incontinent or dead. There seem to be few useful ways to achieve cross-comparisons other than by this mixed panel approach. It is a variant of a widely occurring class of process for resolving legal and other disagreements, whereby the number of **disinterested** parties that can be convinced is taken as an index of the strength of the case.

Despite some progress towards depersonalising the assessed effect of different disabilities on quality of life, it cannot be claimed that efficient and just mechanisms yet exist for allocating health care resources between disciplines or between patient groups on the basis of measured need. Increasing needs in an ageing population, increasing awareness and expectations, and increasing costs from new medical knowledge and technology make inevitable some form of explicit rationing (rather than the present haphazard set of obstacles to access). Even if the absolute total resources put into health care were permitted to rise choices would still have to be faced. As from 1991 this need has become widely and publicly acknowledged[7] although there is no agreement on a basis of rationing that might be widely acceptable. The conceptual and ethical problems remain formidable. The study of health economics is not yet in a position to allow society to distribute resources in a precise way to maximise the health gain per unit of resource. At the policy level, the economic concept of the existing 'burden of disease' (or 'burden of care') is of some use as a multiplier in decisions about the research that might enable prevention or implementation that may improve efficiency. It raises further difficulties in application, when restricted to the costs of formal caring. However this concept begs many important questions about the degree of need and the actual effectiveness of care on the quality of life in those cared for and the quality of life and unquantifiable economic losses to those obliged to care informally (typically daughters).

Table 1.1 illustrates the 'burden of disease' for major disease groups. It would be fallacious to argue that burden of care should be proportional to other economic costs (such as working days lost) or even to some prevalence-weighted index of distress and disability, because allocation of service resources has to depend on effectiveness, i.e. on the improvement in quality of life achieved.

TABLE 1.1 *The burden of disease*

ICD Chapter	Disabled Life Years Kpa (%)	Community Care Costs £m	Other NHS (NHS + CC) £m	Total Costs £m (%)
Mental	98 (10)	1,177·1	2,833·3	4,010·4 (36)
Nervous System	54 (6)	428·6	498·3	926·9 (8)
Eye Complaints	1,343 (14)	457·9	418·8	876·7 (8)
Ear Complaints	2,250 (24)	415·2	388·6	803·8 (7)
Circulatory	1,572 (17)	720·7	1,701·3	2,422·0 (22)
Musculoskeletal	2,815 (30)	1,076·7	988·8	2,065·4 (19)

These figures were compiled and used by the Department of Health for England in 1990 for policy and planning purposes. Among other considerations they contributed to the emphasis upon mental health in 'Health of the Nation' and in the NHS Research and Development programme. Although the figures are composed on the basis of physiological systems, the implications for disability are relatively straightforward: hearing disorders and locomotor disorders top the league for the number of life years affected.

However, the burden of care cannot be ignored unsatisfactory term though it is. Irrespective of the life-destructive qualities of some jobs or the actual need for labour (which is less convincing in times of chronic unemployment or recession) the ability to work is a useful gross proxy for the quality of life. Sensory disabilities may not cost the state much; their prevention or amelioration would have large scope to benefit the economy if the age profile of prevalence were centred on the earlier decades of life. For other non-economic human activities; the ramifications of visual and auditory disabilities are great at all ages.

Despite the intractable issues posed by rationing, there are moves to guide decisions on the implementation of major new programmes according to cost-utility analysis, particularly their ability to maximise the quality-adjusted life-years (QALYs) achieved for each pound spent on health.[8] The total quality-adjusted life-years is the (expected) survival time after a disease or treatment, multiplied by a scaling factor for the degree of disability and hence distress suffered. The health measure has tended to arise from a short hierarchy of items in major areas of disability, distress and dependency rather than the use of the larger questionnaires recommended for surveys and measures of outcomes in trials. However the diffidence about accepting QALYs for widespread use lies deeper. It is certainly problematic to equate a combination of large improvement in the quality of life accompanying short duration with the converse combination, because other contributions to quality of life in a long life are unknown and the effects may not simply be additive. However, few decisions between alternatives would actually involve such extreme trade-offs. The QALY concept is even more difficult to apply in **individual** treatment decisions, explaining why many doctors do not like it. Despite these difficulties in applying the concept quantitatively in practice, there is now much agreement that evidence on degree of need, numbers, achievable benefits, life expectancy and the burden of alternative forms of care should be made available systematically whenever resourcing decisions are made. Whatever the difficulties in its measurement and application, the QALY concept has merit in abstract comparisons for policy in allocating health resources, potentially reducing disagreements by integrating the duration with the quality of life. However, any general agreement to adopt such approaches in purchasing decisions (which has not yet been reached) will not totally remove disagreements, because of the essentially political nature of competition for resources. It is most important to develop and use the essential concept of quality of life, and to stop issues and measurement being avoided on grounds of unease about its full-blown use in the full QALY concept—a more contentious matter.

> *Conclusion: In advanced countries the disabilities are among the major health problems. As this position results in part from past successes of innovations that save lives, it would be logically consistent for those who emphasise high-technology curative life-saving medicine now to shift towards measures of quality of life that fully reflect the disabilities as the major outcome indicator for health programmes in general and for specific treatment regimes.*

4. OVERCOMING THE 'IMAGE' PROBLEM

The necessity for absolute improvements in services for the hearing-impaired became widely recognised in the 1970s. Precisely documenting the **relative** importance of hearing impairment to the quality of extended lives was not required at that time. Although quantification of needs and health gain relative to other disabilities and disease has not so far been required, it may be in the future. Fully complying with that eventual requirement will demand data more relevant and more deliberately acquired than exist in most areas of disease or disability. It is of more immediate relevance to analyse **why** services for the hearing-impaired and other disabled groups had become trapped in a Cinderella status.

Direct advocacy for specific service improvements by sympathetic politicians and by patients' organisations can often be influential. Many of the improvements in research and service for hearing impairment in the UK in the last quarter century have benefited at the national level from the personal involvement of Lord Ashley of Stoke, formerly Jack Ashley, MP. Without his advocacy, several would not have occurred at all. More generally, advocacy for the hearing-impaired is not as widespread as the severity and prevalence warrant, due to much denial and hiding of the socially stigmatised condition of impaired hearing.[9] A second reason for the restricted amount of articulate lobbying has been the dissociation of the occupational impact of hearing impairment from its prevalence. For a given degree of impairment the typical **non**-manual worker is likely to suffer greater obstacles to the pursuit of his work than a manual worker is, because of the greater demands on spoken communication; certainly service uptake is higher in non-manual workers. However, across a range of pathologies, the actual prevalence of impairment is much higher in manual workers.[10] Hence prevalence is dissociated both from the context of maximum occupational impact and from the socio-economic strata that more typically contain decision-makers, pressure groups, opinion-leaders and advocates. Thirdly, audiological services have not benefited much from 'provider push'. By this latter term I mean the tendency for providers of services to marshal support in health authorities and among the public at large for the services that they wish to supply to their patients. As a basis for planning or rationing it has drawbacks, despite its virtue of engaging appropriate activism or professional pride. Only a few members of the senior profession delivering health care to hearing-impaired people, ENT surgeons, have been highly assertive in pioneering and extending at national level the services for the large numbers of hearing-impaired people. This is because the most widely applicable solutions have not generally been surgical solutions that would bring to surgeons the conventional forms of intellectual excitement and prestige. As described in Chapter 5,

the recent advent of cochlear implants (a form of prosthetic rehabilitative management with an important surgical component)
may create a break with this past pattern.

*Conclusion: Understanding and addressing the reasons why the
study and rehabilitation of hearing disorders, and the disabilities
more generally, receive Cinderella status is a pre-requisite to
improving their position.*

5. TERMINOLOGY, DOMAINS AND ATTITUDES IN THE DISABILITIES

The consequences of habitual use of terminology are far-reaching;
one was seen in the consultative document for future health policy
produced by the UK government in the summer of 1991, *Health
of the Nation*. Although the penultimate draft proposed the rehabilitation of the 'physical' disabilities as a priority area, the final
document omitted rehabilitation and disability as a priority target
for population health measures. (It subsequently emerged as a
priority area for the NHS Research and Development Programme.) The wording and the evident epidemiological context
suggested that there was no specific intention to exclude sight and
hearing from 'physical', but all the examples were drawn from
locomotor disabilities. Hearing, much more than sight, carries
contact with the social world rather than with the physical (i.e.
spatial and mechanical) world, so the inclusion of hearing disability with locomotor disorders would seem to rest uneasily with past
common usage of 'disability', which has mostly meant locomotor
disability. The term 'hearing **disability**' used professionally to
convey an intended distinction of domain, (i.e. contrasting with
the impairment domain) therefore seems strange to the non-ini-
tiated, whereas the term 'hearing impairment' has now become
fairly conventional. Yet a sensory disability (although appropriately studied in a sub-branch of the neurosciences) would indeed
be considered by most lay people and by psychologists to be a
sub-class of physical (i.e. bodily) disability, in contrast to a psychological (i.e. cognitive or interpersonal) disability. Leaving aside
issues of terminology among the general public, large discrepan-
cies in terminology exist between different professional groups.
Because of the historical view of development as a competition,

psychologists, educationists and others with a developmental per-spective have tended to refer to 'handicapped children' without intending any distinction of domain.[11] So there is need for some order among these usages.

A major obstacle to clarity lies in the refusal of all these terms referring to impairment, disability or handicap to stand still; a term introduced deliberately to avoid stigma may within 20 years be thought by some to have become stigmatising and in turn be displaced. Currently the term 'physically challenged' is being promoted to replace 'disabled', and the formerly mild and non-specific connotations of learning disabilities have moved to cover those not capable of a totally independent life. At the purposive level the concept of a challenge is appropriate, and it may even be useful in (re)habilitation. However it is a logical error to substitute a purposive term where a general descriptive one is required. In such examples the advocate's political correctness is publicised at the price of much confusion, then ridiculed by tabloid columnists. To reject the term 'disabled' as stigmatising is to misallocate faults in humanity (competitiveness and stigmatisation) onto the descriptive term itself. These logical errors on the part of advocates supply a continuous downwards motion to the terms that researchers and health care professionals would prefer were stationary. Confusion arises because distinctions are required that the revisions are not designed to achieve.

Not all innovation in terms is unproductive; it can be well thought out, as in the *WHO International Classification of Impairment, Disability and Handicap.*[12] In 1981, shortly after the publication of this terminology I was giving a talk at a large district general hospital that serves the Fenlands, an isolated agricultural corner of England; I used the now common general term 'hearing impairment'. This term amazed and amused my audience, particularly the general practitioners in it. They plainly thought the term not one designed to convey some necessary conceptual distinction of domain, but yet another unnecessary euphemism. They could perhaps be pardoned for thinking that 'deafness' an Anglo-Saxon word of which a close equivalent has served Fenland well for 1,400 years was adequate to embrace any loss of hearing, from a temporary dullness following a cold, through to the total absence of auditory response. However, the matter is not quite so simple, as the allocation of professional effort does require distinctions to be made. 'Impairment' **is** a useful general term for organ dysfunction, and is not (in the way that my audience supposed), an instance of euphemistic terminologial leap-frogging to escape stigmatisation. However a reaction to instances of leap-frogging is mounting. No less a columnist than Nigella Lawson (*London Evening Standard*, 16 October 1991), in an otherwise very apt tirade against self-defeating euphemisms of American origin, mistook 'hard-of-hearing' for an euphemism. In fact, the long-established vernacular term 'hard-of-hearing' exists to make one of the major distinctions required; the term primarily refers to moderate late-acquired losses of hearing. The tendency to reject some valuable new distinctions as tendentious is also widespread among professionals: but the occurrence of neologistic excesses does not entitle us to ignore real distinctions.

The terms 'impairment', 'disability' and 'handicap' are distinguished by their derivation in English, and now internationally by definition. They should not be used to refer to different degrees in the same domain (although sloppy usage occasionally implies that) but to different domains. The degrees of impairment, disability and handicap are substantially inter-correlated. The correlation is imperfect, because as we move successively between domains in the pre-dominant causal sequence of pathology⇒impairment⇒disability⇒handicap, various extra determinants such as individual adjustment also enter. Impairment is essentially the loss of function in a system of the body, although the WHO usage subsumes in impairment the structural abnormality (pathology) underlying that loss.

Impairment, as a loss of organ function, is the linking domain between disability and pathology, the latter being the anatomical manifestation of disease. Impairment measures are often used to anchor observations in other domains. Impairment is also usually the domain most readily used to quantify severity within an area, because it is most amenable to calibrated quantitative measurement. In hearing, the loss of organ function is usually represented by the loss of sensitivity to faint sounds, because this measure is widely predictive of other attributes of concern. Disability is the inability to perform useful basic activities or functions of the whole person (e.g. walking, accurately perceiving speech sounds, etc) that the environment may demand in various contexts and forms. The need to exercise a distinction between impairment and disability in hearing has been reduced by their obviously high correlation, due in turn to the basic abilities depending on only a limited number of aspects of a physiological system. However the ability to walk depends upon adequate functioning of the respiratory, cardiovascular, muscular, neural and joint systems; this illustrates the need for the distinction.

Disability is essentially absolute and is essentially a performance concept, referring to normal and useful capacities that an individual lacks. However, the practical difficulties of obtaining broad-based performance measures of disability that entail surrogate measures, either cross-predictions from impairment measures, or self-reports of disability (including the emotional reaction to having the disability) are typically used for most purposes, instead of true disability measures; thus conflicting concepts of what disability is have grown up. The choice of a general chapter-heading word to refer to a particular area in discussions of **all** its domains (impairment, disability or handicap) remains problematic. 'Disorder' is sometimes used in this way, but that is also sometimes used to refer to the underlying pathophysiology; 'impairment' is becoming increasingly common for this purpose. Many European languages lack a set of terms that can be readily aligned with the WHO terms based on English etymology and specific usages; this will continue to be an obstacle to international communication for many years.

It is possible for an impairment to lead to a handicap, without there being any evident disability, e.g. in the case of a disfigurement. Handicap is essentially socio-economic and relative, referring to the social and economic disadvantages suffered as a consequence of the impairment and disability. Because of its popular sporting associations, handicap is perhaps subject to less conceptual confusion than disability in its concrete everyday usage. However, as a domain variable it is multi-determined and hence even less predictable and more difficult to measure in individuals, because of the greater scope for individuals' aspirations and for families' attitudes to influence actual achievement in the longer term. It is notable that the WHO terminology which has proved useful for positivist science is unpopular among disabled people and their advocates.

In any measurement of health status or morbidity, there is a classical opposition between objective and subjective definitions.

Clinical observations are often informal and intuitively guided so do not provide a prime example of objectivity; they are often mis-allocated as the 'objective' pole in this opposition, contrasting with reports of symptoms and satisfaction (or otherwise), which provide the prime examples of subjective indicators. Protagonists in debates about appropriate outcome measures occasionally state an extreme subjectivist or objectivist view—perhaps just to annoy their adversaries. The patient's perception of his own problem certainly has great implications as a major determinant of behaviour in seeking help, and of regarding help as having been effectively given. Professionals who do not take this into account, including asking directly about it, will tend to end up giving ineffective, low quality services; but this is an issue in delivery, not one in deciding on whether what is delivered is effective in ways that can be publicly justified. It is important to register that my emphasis on objectivity builds on a definition of 'objective' as including any systematic observation in which qualities and quantities are verifiable. This by no means rules out performance tests and voluntary behaviours, which are often in the medical context incorrectly denoted 'subjective', in contrast with involuntary behaviours such as reflexes. The extreme view that **only** the patient's view of his symptom and satisfaction matters—even if qualified to apply to the longer term—is a signpost away from medicine to quackery, for example via the over-use of placebos. I therefore maintain that impairment, disability and handicap are all essentially objective concepts, despite difficulties in their objective measurement, and that treatment or remediation should be measured objectively wherever this is possible. Subjective processes may influence behaviour and even the objective indicators of outcomes. The process of adjustment is an important example of this subjective mediation; psychosomatic medicine provides others. Subjective measures may provide adequate, even relevant, surrogate indicators. They are also of practical importance and should be provided for in a supplementation of the WHO definitions, not by a perversion of them.

Conclusion: There is good reason to allow development of technical terms for the disabilities beyond those of common usage, provided that the modifications are driven by the systematic need for useful distinctions among objective measures rather than by fashion and euphemism. The WHO terminology of impairment, disability and handicap makes useful distinctions without the artificiality of neologism. The concepts are essentially objective but a set of subjective concepts and terms is also required.

6. ADJUSTMENT AS A PRODUCT OF EXPERIENCE AND CULTURE

Adjustment is an unstable balance between striving to overcome disability and the acceptance of it. Even without the confounding created by individuals' personalities and attitudes, the natural reduction of expectations with ageing makes it difficult and time-consuming to obtain reliable measures of a person's social functioning (for example, to measure the consequences of an impairment of hearing or language and to evaluate interventions). Unless a person's deterioration of hearing has been sudden and recent, a questionnaire may under-estimate the degree of social isolation, because adjustments have occurred and expectations have long been lowered. This under-estimation obviously creates a difficulty in verbal responses to questionnaires, but it also occurs with observations of behaviour.

Whilst 'hearing-impaired' can be a mouthful, the term 'deaf' in popular usage has several meanings. It is losing (albeit slowly) the associations that used to make hearing-impaired people the butt of music-hall jokes. Among those that consider themselves to be 'deaf', the word is used in two main, loosely aligned, ways: (i) absence of any functionally useful hearing, i.e. the presence of a degree of impairment in the profound-total range; (ii) membership of a community in which sign language, not speech, is the prime mode of interpersonal communication. Members of the signing deaf community feel that they are insufficiently understood by society at large, and that in some respects they deserve a better deal. Although they feel 'apart' and in some respects excluded, in most contexts they do not nowadays feel marginalised or stigma-tised in the way that some of the severely hard-of-hearing do, precisely because they constitute the majority in their own distinct social world. Among the signing deaf community, the word 'deaf' expresses a very positive identity. Had some of its members been present at my talk mentioned in the previous section, they would not have been happy at the rural GPs (some of whom had never met a member of this community) borrowing and applying the label 'deaf' so widely. The most serious identity problem is met in those who become severely or profoundly impaired in adolescence or adult life, yet who cannot through geographical isolation be part of the separate deaf community, or who do not wish to be; many of these people do feel excluded and stigmatised in addition to the obvious stresses in, and practical limitations upon, their lives. Thus, in the handicap domain in particular, a graded terminology for the effects of hearing impairment is essential, which reflects the categorical distinctions and gradations amongst the various groups with differing modes of adjustment, whose attitudes to the evolving terminology and usage are also different.

Differing adjustments generate widely differing perspectives. As an extreme example, normally-hearing parents may view with alarm the prospect of having a deaf child; given the possibility of being unable to communicate with him or her, they might even consider this prospect to be grounds for the termination of a pregnancy in which the probability of severe deafness is high. However, to already deaf parents the prospect of a deaf child is unremarkable, and more practical problems might even be anticipated in their making full provision for a hearing child. Outsiders to professional work with deaf and hearing-impaired people (and indeed many insiders) do not appreciate that these two viewpoints are simply irreconcilable. Both have to be noted by the professional or scientist working in this field, but debate, proselytisation or attempts to impose one set of values upon those who hold the other set are futile. As one practical consequence, any offer of reproductive choice to parents would have to be phrased in very general, abstract (hence, unfortunately, rather wordy) terms, so as to avoid making value judgements that only the particular parents-to-be themselves can make. The growing prospects for primary prevention by genetic counselling, briefly reviewed in Chapter 5, inevitably increase the tension between the two viewpoints. I have very little to say in what follows about 'the signing deaf', but I have used this conflict of perspectives to illustrate the diversity of categories of hearing-impaired person from which a diversity of service provision necessarily flows. As an example outside the health sphere, several tens of thousands of people can benefit from signed programmes or inset sign-language interpretation on television, and many more benefit from the sub-titling of a few programmes. However, repeated attempts to persuade producers of television and radio comedy and drama to reduce the level of sound-effects relative to speech have so far been unsuccessful. Although this would benefit millions, it threatens the artistic view of the mainstream product and is less readily associated with the popular charitable impulse to provide some readily acknowledged special facilities for a labelled minority.

There is a point beyond which treatment of the pathology or even the secondary prevention of disability becomes decreasingly relevant; emphasis has at that point to switch to enhancing an individual's coping strategy, and manipulating the psychological framework plus the social and educational environment in an adaptive way, so as to minimise the socio-economic and personal disadvantage or handicap that it brings. This adjustment often has to involve some degree of acceptance of the impairment and disability. Severity of the impairment can contribute to determining where the switch point between these two emphases is located, but timing and reversibility also contribute. To the rare individual who has irretrievably lost all his hearing, neither an understanding of the anatomy of the ear and related spaces and tissues in the head, nor an understanding of auditory psychophysics underpins much professional help. To the millions whose hearing is imperfect, the consequences of both types of study are high relevant. Not all affected individuals fall neatly in all respects on one or other side of the dividing point where this emphasis has to switch; around this point there are major ambiguities of perspective, tensions of individual identity, shifts of professional responsibility and of scientific grouping. A preventable or treatable condition has to be viewed as an eradicable mistake of nature; a person with an inescapable condition cannot view it thus, but must see it as a challenge for adjustment—determining the right balance between insistence on legislated universal rights of access, striving to compensate, and the acceptance of limitations.

> *Conclusion: Acceptance of the disabled state when there is no alternative confers a singular perspective on the world. In profound deafness this involves coping with great stress, and great isolation, or else entry into a distinct sub-culture with its own social categories.*

7. RELEVANCE OF 'THE MEDICAL MODEL'

When grouping problems of hearing together with problems of sight or locomotion, for example, we talk about 'disablement' or the 'disabilities'. One reason for assuming any such grouping is a possible similarity of the rehabilitative approach apparently required in the appropriate forms of professional action for the various disabilities. Where **counselling** for adjustment may be involved, an obviously greater similarity exists than any similarity of pharmaceutical treatments for heterogeneous diseases; however it is not quite so obvious that **re-training** or use of compensatory strategies to reduce or offset disability in performance permits an approach to be used that is similar in detailed ways for hearing and vision. Except at the most general level the principle of re-learning research to explore such similarities systematically has not been done. Indeed, there has been rather little research on processes of re-learning and adjustment or on how these can be facilitated.

In Western countries, a conceptual grouping of the disabilities is sometimes seen at the level of research or legislation and occasionally in the founding of multi-problem welfare agencies, but only rarely. Blind people do not appreciate being classed with deaf people nor *vice versa*; such a failure to make a distinction of both practical and ideological importance may in part underlie the feeling that super-ordinate terms such as 'disabled' are stigmatising. There has never been a serious movement in the UK to place the provision of care for different groups of disabled people under one agency or (para-medical) profession. Nor within the health sphere has there been any major move to favour a wholly behavioural model; this would mean abandoning the medical model of care delivery that is rooted in the institutionalised division of medicine into disciplines that are based mostly on the location and form of pathology or impairment. Such a recombination could be envisaged in research and it might have some benefits in bringing greater theoretical coherence, and more expert direction and evaluation into the work of the diverse rehabilitative professions allied to medicine. However, persuading institutions to combine is hard in the best of circumstances, and a major scientific synthesis and progress based on a general applied psychology of the disabilities would probably have to be a prerequisite for foreseeing any such union. Attempts to discuss all the disabilities together, or at least an equivalent, have been largely restricted to social scientists using the interpretative approach (Section 2 above) based on a set of categories derived from the study of ethnic discrimination. This has given some useful insights, but it is not yet clear that it has led to much concrete progress. I see a 'marriage' type of re-organisation of the professions serving the disabilities as unlikely.

A second type of re-organisation integrating the disabilities could come from another quarter altogether—economic pressures. One reason for considering the disabilities as a whole is the immense population need for simple forms of rehabilitation at the primary care level. This need could only be met by some form of generic primary rehabilitation worker with a limited repertoire of techniques, relatively little responsibility for assessment and referral to secondary or tertiary centres, but a large role in after-care for those discharged from secondary or tertiary centres. In turn this would require more hierarchical professional structures, with higher levels of academic achievement, research involvement, professional achievement and managerial responsibility at the top than currently exists in the relatively flat career structures of many medical and paramedical professions for example dentistry and speech therapy.

Within the framework of medical disciplines, rehabilitation of the disabilities is relatively new and receives only modest interest, resources and status; it is something of an after-thought to the diagnosis and treatment of the underlying pathology. Ideally, rehabilitation itself would be a leading discipline but there are currently only four medical chairs of rehabilitation in the UK. Four realities make it likely that work based on an acceptance of a modified medical model will be more effective in the near future than work based on its abandonment: (i) Absence of a theoretical framework and of evaluation studies leaves some uncertainty about the extent and routine of the benefits that rehabilitation can deliver, in terms of measurable impact. (In fairness, questioning the efficacy of accepted regimes of medical and surgical treatment is equally necessary.) (ii) As noted earlier, publicly expressed attitudes are proving slow to shift from a concern with death and acute illness to quality of survival. (iii) At the same time as new, and in some instances expensive, opportunities are opening up for effective treatment in some areas of medicine, the bottled-up demand for relatively simple forms of rehabilitation and care for chronic problems, chiefly in the ageing population, is increasingly seen as limitless; real resources available have not been growing sufficiently to meet the growth in total need. It is therefore not clear that growth and development in the rehabilitation of disabilities will be permitted to occur on a scale, that might justify or enable any wholesale re-organisation towards generic rehabilitation workers in the near future. (A vertical restructuring is perhaps not to be ruled out). (iv) A major institutional shift towards grouping of professions by effects rather than causes, and a shift of responsibility within the health sphere to a rehabilitative agency, bridging all areas of disability and emphasising skill training and adjustment, might discourage attempts at prevention of disabilities. A medical (disease-based) model does at least link primary, secondary and tertiary prevention with rehabilitation in each area. Thus, while my preventive stance and my partly behavioural orientation lead me to recommend increased flexibility in applying the medical model, I do not favour replacing it outright.

Conclusion: Promotion of rehabilitation and adjustment in disability and handicap is valuable, but should not take place at the expense of prevention and treatment of disease and impairment.

8. MODES OF INTERVENTION

There are five modes of intervention in which health services may be judged as effective or otherwise: primary prevention; secondary prevention; tertiary prevention; palliation; and rehabilitation. Actual 'packages' of care, even for the limited range of individual patients receiving a single diagnostic label, will often embrace several of these modes. It is useful to characterise current services by their present distribution of these modes; equally, forecasting requires assessment of the potential for improvement in each mode in the future, based on current trends in fundamental knowledge. Primary prevention is total prevention in the layperson's sense, exemplified by cutting out exposure or undermining pathogenicity (quarantine, not smoking, protective clothing, etc.). In secondary prevention timing of intervention influences the quality of outcome; it is best thought of as assurance of the least adverse of a range of possible outcomes, by shifting or reversing a state which, from its general known natural history, would progress or be compounded adversely with time. Because secondary prevention is particularly important in development and in hearing I return to it below. Tertiary prevention embraces much conventional treatment which does not reverse or arrest **progression** in a time-bound way (and is hence not true prevention), but which attenuates the severity of a condition subsequently or shortens its duration; urgency may be desirable but does not influence outcome. The distinction between secondary and tertiary prevention can be subtle, and is made even more complicated by the fact that both concepts are relevant both to disease and disability. The use of screening or other methods of active case-finding is not a logically defining characteristic of secondary prevention; indeed, removing a diseased appendix is not a sequel of screening but could qualify as secondary prevention. However, because averting progression from asymptomatic to symptomatic status seems more like true prevention than does reactively intervening in acute deterioration, there is a tendency for screening and secondary prevention to be associated.

The widespread necessity for the palliation mode (symptom suppression) may look disappointing in the context of increasingly scientific and technological medicine, but it is a vital ingredient in the effective integration of elements of medical or paramedical practice. A good example of integration of palliation with the other modes occurs in contemporary audiology. My colleague Dr Ross Coles has developed an integrated range of service elements in a specialising clinic for people with tinnitus (the often exasperating buzzing or ringing in the ears so frequently associated with a hearing impairment). This clinic model has evolved over a dozen years, along with the evaluation and optimisation of particular complementary procedures with it. The model[13] involves a diagnostic sequence with systematic consideration of surgical, medical, prosthetic, psychological (rehabilitative) and palliative options, in a sequence determined by assessments and by the apparent success or otherwise of the options exercised up to each option point.

To some, secondary prevention may appear to fall unimpressively between the more remarkable modes of treatment and primary prevention. In terms of the palpable effects of treatment that do not need large-scale trials to verify, tertiary prevention via reactive treatment can appear more impressive to patients or their families whose anxieties have already been raised by a symptomatic condition, than the mere arresting of otherwise progressive conditions which may be asymptomatic. Furthermore, a qualitative argument for not delaying treatment in any condition can already be sustained on the grounds that the total quality of a life accumulated over time will always be improved somewhat by a treatment occurring sooner rather than later (tertiary intervention). The public health issue is the degree of **additional** benefit to the long-term level of functioning considered against the **additional** cost and risks from early case-finding that is followed by intervention. It could be difficult to justify even the research investment required to quantify the specific extra benefits of secondary prevention; well-controlled evidence for a general natural history of progression or compounding of the particular condition may be lacking as may good evidence for the general efficacy of an intervention designed to arrest it. Hence it may be quite difficult to obtain evidence justifying early identification and intervention on the basis of secondary prevention. An objective rather than subjective view of health gain is necessary, to represent fairly the benefits of primary and secondary prevention. If secondary prevention does appear less impressive and more problematic than the other modes, it may seem perverse for me to concentrate upon it in what follows. However, to the medical scientist looking for ways to increase health gain, secondary prevention poses scientific challenges; it has a central position in treatment strategies for hearing impairments, as we shall see. Depending on the magnitude of progression or compounding of the disease in question, secondary prevention effects may be substantially larger than tertiary prevention effects. Western 20th-century attitudes to fate and opportunity, in the context of the rationing of health care via waiting-lists, can make claims of secondary prevention appear much more impressive in quantitative terms of health gain than mere claims of timeliness—hence, for example, the existence of priority systems for urgent hospital appointments. Secondary prevention can also, if the intervention occurs early in life, receive a large multiplier from the long life expectancy, and hence be convincing in relative terms, for example in QALY comparisons.

Any judgement about the relative importance and promise of

particular modes such as secondary prevention has to be given a 'use-by' date. When I first outlined a research programme for hearing disorders in 1976 neither primary prevention nor medical treatment as a sub-category of tertiary prevention seemed to offer either great possibilities for progress or great likelihood of the availability of the chief forms of resource necessary to pursue the research. I thus opted for a mixture of long-term research towards goals in surgical and prosthetic management with an emphasis upon application in the secondary prevention mode, including the gingering up of services via the epidemiology of need. Developments in biomedical science are now making the prospects for progress in treatment and in primary prevention somewhat better.

> *Conclusion: The idea of early intervention to stop disease, impairment and disability deteriorating (secondary prevention) is of far-reaching importance in otology and audiology.*

9. TIME SCALES

My final two points are not specific to the disabilities, but are of general importance in applicable research. Whatever the influence of the political outlook of any particular era, the hurried policy agendas of 4-to-5 year governments do not make it easy to do and to apply research that is both scientifically pervasive **and** relevant to the currently available or offered policy options. Even with large resources, worthwhile research takes time, so the two requirements stand in tension. For reasons of methodology and training, development projects in clinical research and health services research often have a time-scale of about five years; the interval from conception to application is usually much longer than this and much longer than anticipated. For example, at the present rate of development it is unlikely that **mass** neonatal screening for hearing impairment with the technique of oto-acoustic emissions (see Chapter 3) could be widespread in the UK before 1997 and even targetted (at-risk) screening will not cover all maternity hospitals by that date. Two decades of research and development will have then separated the fundamental discovery from its fullest application, although the general potential in screening could be discerned at the start. The delay has not been due to inertia or to restrictive practices by the scientists involved, who would have liked to have been able to move faster and would individually have received more acclaim had they done so. Rather, there are constraints of finance and organisation and intrinsic limitations set by the progressively more detailed questions requiring answers in the implementation of a technique. How then can policy of governments with a 4-to-5 year time-scale, or the often shorter duration of initiatives of a particular health minister, do any more than edge forward with projects that seem intuitively, and on the best advice at the time, to offer high promise, or to contribute to long-term goals? If taken centrally, decisions on the next stage or on eventual wholesale implementation will fall to other governments or ministers. In appraising options for implementation, the increasing emphasis upon measurement of outcomes makes this tension of time-scale even greater, as many health outcomes become clear only in the longer term. An example of this was seen in the delayed finding of late failures in knee- and hip-joint replacement operations, for which a consensus on a highly favourable balance of cost and benefit with low risk had emerged quite quickly. This consensus subsequently had to be modified as long-term problems developed, although it is still highly favourable in QALY terms. This tension of time-scale is important in scientific advice to government ministers, so that the true stage of the science can be dovetailed with the appropriate stage of policy formation in decisions on research, development, and implementation. The stage of the science and its practical import should neither be oversold (thereby creating premature expectations) nor undersold to interpose unnecessary 'research' as a smoke-screen for inaction.

I do not wish here to force a false opposition between pure and applied science when determining a distinction between short- and long-term views of a sequence of work. One reason that a distinction is difficult to sustain is that time-scale to application is too unstable to provide a defining characteristic. For example in the late 1970s we thought my colleagues' research on hereditary deafness, touched on in Chapter 5, had an application horizon of 20–30 years. The technology of molecular biology has shortened this estimate dramatically; in terms of character and discipline the work remains 'basic' but it is now becoming coupled to clinical research with an application horizon of about five years.

Conclusion: In applicable research, short-term and long-term studies work best as a partnership on a continuum, with mutual involvement; an over-view of their interleaving is crucial.

10. BALANCE IN RESEARCH STRATEGIES

My introduction so far has emphasised the pull of human need more than the push of scientific and technological possibility. However, it is unproductive in the long term, and overall, if too high a percentage of research effort is too closely geared to particular goals formulated in terms of currently perceived needs. It is not widely appreciated **why** a balance is required. Firstly, if a particular envisaged application does not result successfully, nothing may be gained at all, because the issue which the application or technical development embodies is usually highly specific. Secondly, basic knowledge is always potentially informative (in the sense of the mathematical theory of information) because it retains some generality. It is usually acquired in steps (research hypotheses) which are posed in such a way that the answer is neither so likely as to be wastefully redundant, nor so unlikely (over-specific) as to be a reckless gamble. Thirdly, an evolving basic research capacity is an option or a facility developed or preserved; for example in the 1980s UK applied research on AIDS got off to a good start because of existing basic work on retroviruses.

The reason why curiosity-led research is valuable has a formal mathematical basis, but can be appreciated intuitively via an analogy, as follows. You are driving to a destination near the centre of a large city; do you not know it well, but you have some idea of the relationship between landmarks in and around the centre. Once in the congested centre you have to face traffic jams or perhaps pay a street mileage charge introduced by the City Council to combat jams and pollution. It is hence likely that the quickest or cheapest way to your destination is not the most direct route by the map, particularly if the destination is not on the approach side of the central area. Even if you do not have an exact near-optimal route in mind, it is worth some speculative or even circuitous driving on the faster open suburban roads until you reach a sector which you know will give you a short final route into your destination. This is a valid analogy because in research and development the final path (development for routine application and production engineering, in an industrial context) is usually very expensive. An example outside the health sphere is building a pilot manufacturing plant that can only operate in a limited number of ways. In the health sphere we see the same principle in the high overheads of organising a model service or a large multi-centre trial with uniform procedures. Relatively modest resources can be usefully expended in a wide search for progress across a broad front, but the number of highly expensive final paths to be tried out in the development stage close to final routine application has to be kept as few as possible. The distribution of effort overall will be most cost-effective if the structure is genuinely oriented towards a search for applicable ideas, facts and principles. This requires a clear recognition of what is likely to be a productive step towards a worthwhile application goal. This goal orientation has not always been present in past basic research, and the skills in the recognition of applicability could probably be better taught than they are. However, there is increasing realisation[14] in the academic study of science policy that major searches and surges of basic research activity are indeed driven by at least broad visions of applicability, such as the lucrative prospects from commercial patenting of a cure for cancer or a room-temperature superconductor.

The search model with emphasis on early-stage activity (fast suburban driving, on the analogy) should not be misconstrued as an argument favouring 'knowledge for knowledge's sake'. That unfortunate expression is generally unhelpful, and leads to a widespread misunderstanding that basic research is the satisfaction of idle curiosity. Freed of the misunderstanding about knowledge for knowledge's sake, many of the arguments about pure *versus* applied research, basic *versus* development work, etc. simply disappear. They can be replaced by more detailed discussions of: (i) the set of particular goals; (ii) the tapering of many inexpensive basic research projects into a few expensive applied projects, and (iii) the maintenance of the facilities (in the broadest sense, including perspectives, training opportunities, classes of technique, and whole disciplines) that will best undertake different parts of the searches.

Conclusion: Good applied research is difficult to do; it is especially difficult to choose well the few large projects that can be afforded.

Commitment of the usual necessary large resources should only be made when the pointers from a wide range of information, mostly from more basic research, are distinctly favourable. Basic research can be curiosity-driven, but the curiosity should not be idle.

This chapter has discussed some issues in policy for implementation, and in the initiation and conduct of science in general. Reflection upon the dynamics and direction of research and development is quite common where 'big science' and its role in the national economy are concerned. It is much less common in the health sphere and particularly in the disability field. Without the insights offered by such reflection, the appropriate direction and the potential or limitations of research may be misunderstood not merely by the public and politicians, but also by professionals quite close to the research.

REFERENCES

1. PARKER, G., AND BALDWIN, S., (1992). 'Confessions of a jobbing researcher'. *Disability and Society*, **7**(2), 197–203.
2. OLIVER, M., 'Changing the social relations of research production?' *Disability and Society*, **7**(2), 101–114.
3. COLVEZ, A., AND BLANCHET, M., (1983). 'Potential gains in life expectancy free of disability: a tool for health planning'. *International Journal of Epidemiology*, **12**(2), 224–229.
4. BEBBINGTON, A. C., (1988). 'The expectation of life without disability in England and Wales'. *Social Science in Medicine*, **27**(4), 321–326.
5. ROBINE, J. M., AND RITCHIE, K., (1991). 'Healthy life expectancy: evaluation of global indicator of change in population health'. *British Medical Journal*, **302**, 457–460.
6. MARTIN, J., MELTZER, H., AND ELLIOT, D., (1988). *The prevalence of disability among adults*. OPCS, London.
7. COCHRANE, M., HAM, C., HEGINBOTHAM, C., AND SMITH, R., (1991). 'Rationing: at the cutting edge'. *British Medical Bulletin*, **303**, 1039–1042.
8. WILLIAMS, A., (1985). 'Economics of coronary artery by-pass grafting'. *British Medical Journal*, **291**, 326–329.
9. HUMPHREY, C., GILHOME-HERBST, K., AND FARUQI, S., (1980). 'Some characteristics of the hearing-impaired elderly who do not present themselves for rehabilitation'. *British Journal of Audiology*, **15**, 25–30.
10. DAVIS, A. C., (1989). 'The prevalence of hearing impairment and reported hearing disability among adults in Great Britain'. *International Journal of Epidemiology*, **18**(4), 911–917.
11. HAGGARD, M. P., (1985). 'Concepts of impairment disability and handicap'. *Bulletin of the British Psychological Society*, **38**, 83.

12. WORLD HEALTH ORGANISATION (1980). *International classification of impairments, disabilities and handicaps*. WHO, Geneva.

13. JENSEN, J. H., (1990). 'Presbyacusis and other age-related aspects'. *Proceedings of 14th Danavox Symposium*: Danavox Jubilee Foundation, Copenhagen: ISBN 87–982422–3–7, 377–402.

14. TURNEY, J., (1991). 'What drives the engines of innovation?' *New Scientist*, **132**(1795), 35–40.

2

HEARING: SOME USEFUL AUDIOLOGICAL CONCEPTS

THE ISSUES RAISED IN CHAPTER 1 WERE GENERAL; FOR EXAMPLE, areas other than hearing have problems of terminology. However, the point was established that in order to appreciate current needs for specific services for hearing impairment and disability, we need further factual background on hearing and its disorders. Full appreciation of issues in research and development towards new services require even more grounding, but I will restrict this short tutorial chapter to a few perspectives that specifically advance the exposition of the main chapters where further detail and implications for services will be pursued. Up-to-date texts are available, both elementary[1] and advanced.[2]

Hearing relies on a chain of biological processes, each of which can be affected by disease. As well as local trauma or infection, various systemic diseases of brain, bone and blood, and of functionally connected but distant organs such as the kidney, can all affect the integrity of the auditory system. However, there can be difficulties in interpreting the core pathology in a particular disease as **causing** all associated raised risks of hearing impairment. Many such reported associations are spurious, due to the adoption of over-select controls, which fail to reflect the generally high prevalence of mild hearing impairment. Also, clinical samples with one problem tend to have generally raised prevalence of other problems compared to their population peers. It is still wise to view the causation of hearing impairment as diverse and multifactorial, and not to jump to conclusions about individuals who also have specific diseases of other organs. With the exception of a few well-defined conditions this makes the attribution of a single or definite cause in the individual difficult. This predicament is unfortunately a poor stimulus to the emergence of a strong

References begin on p. 42.

professional framework of diagnosis and treatment; research and development towards genuine diagnosis in hearing disorders according to cause require deliberate encouragement. Meanwhile, a balance has to be carefully judged between investing in high-risk research that may enable such discoveries (and hence ultimately revolutionise prevention or treatment), *versus* investing in a lower-risk style of research that is likely to improve practice in respects that may be individually modest, although cumulatively worthwhile in terms of health gain.

The two applied problem areas covered in the following chapters have drawn heavily upon fundamental research—for example, products of earlier research became part of the procedures or instrumentation in service delivery and there is still room in each for radical advances to improve practice. However the areas were originally chosen on a low-risk strategy because the prospects for worthwhile advances in the near future seemed good. The two areas are (i) hearing disorders in children and (ii) the highly prevalent progressive mild-to-moderate impairments of middle and old age. Area (i) sub-divides into: (a) the detection and treatment of highly prevalent (but fluctuating and eventually remitting) middle-ear disease in young children, with particular reference to the oto-pathological and cognitive sequelae; and (b) the early detection and (re)habilitation of congenital severe and profound hearing impairments. In terms of prevalences, age ranges, natural history and pathogenesis of the diseases, the conditions in areas (i) and (ii) could hardly appear more disparate. Yet there are three important similarities. The first similarity is the appropriate mode of intervention which for the foreseeable future is largely restricted to secondary and tertiary prevention of disability. The opportunities for primary prevention and for effective curative treatment, although not totally absent, remain very limited. The second similarity lies in the fact that the people most affected are at the extremes of the age range and not breadwinners—those under 6 and those over 60 years. The extreme age ranges also tend to experience high miscellaneous morbidity, by comparison with the distinct sources of economically significant morbidity or mortality occurring in mid-late adulthood, such as cardiovascular disease. Diseases of bread-winners are more frequently the focus of powerful disease-specific pressure groups and research charities, or of active health promotion campaigns.

The third similarity is the difficulty of talking sense about service delivery in each instance without a clear grasp of the prevalence/ severity distribution. This concept ought to be familiar, but probably requires introduction.

1. THE PREVALENCE/SEVERITY DISTRIBUTION

Hearing impairment is a matter of degree. Hearing loss, or more precisely the hearing threshold level (HTL), is measured in decibels (dB). Mathematically the decibel is ten times (deci-) the logarithm of the power ratio (-bel) between the sound in question and some specific reference sound. Here the reference is a sound just intense enough for a healthy otologically screened young person to hear it under physically and psychophysically defined conditions. The standard scientific and clinical way to measure hearing impairment is as the sound pressure level (SPL) necessary to just hear single-frequency tones at a range of standard frequencies, i.e. the sound pressure at threshold. HTL values are closely related to, although not identical to, the familar SPL values attributing, for example, to a busy street a typical value of 80 dB SPL. The HTL is a quantity in the impairment domain; because the threshold is the minimum audible sound, increasing impairments have increasing positive HTLs. However, it is customary in a clinical context to plot increasing positive, i.e. 'worse' values downwards on a chart known as the audiogram (FIG. 2.1).

This method of definition of hearing impairment has for over 50 years withstood attempts to supplant it, partly because of its useful scale properties. The numerical values which result correspond closely to intuitive judgements of the percentage disability suffered in the commoner (cochlear) type of hearing impairment. Various scales for medico-legal assessment of 'disability' have generally used surrogate impairment measures with only minor modifications to the dB HTL scale, for an appropriate set of frequencies. Over the range in hearing thresholds seen in patients commonly encountered, the auditory disabilities resulting from the two main types of impairment (conductive, cochlear) are comparable. This holds true only for normal-to-loud speech; for highly amplified speech, conductive hearing losses lead to lesser auditory disability, whereas for quiet speech cochlear losses have the advantage.

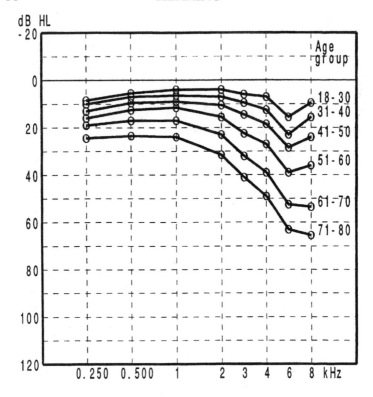

FIGURE 2.1 This figure illustrates the audiogram, the standard clinical graphic representation of data on auditory sensitivity, which provide the most widely used type of test of hearing organ function. Hearing threshold level is plotted down the ordinate, log frequency along the abscissa. The 'baseline' at the top is the International Standard derived from samples of otologically screened normal young adults. Clinically up to four curves for one individual would be plotted, with symbols distinguishing left from right ears, and air-from bone-conduction. The given curves plotted are mean HTL values for decade age groups in the contemporary British population (better ear data). Three points can be illustrated: (i) actual young adults hear appreciably less well than the standard; (ii) the typical middle-aged or elderly person has a high-frequency hearing loss; (iii) subject to considerations of differential mortality hearing losses appear to accelerate with age.

The terminological distinction between people who are 'cases' of hearing impairment and those who are not, does not correspond to a biological dichotomy. It displays a continuous distribution, which I denote 'the prevalence/severity distribution' of which examples are given in later chapters. The sub-distribution of prevalence/severity for various categories of hearing impairment according to cause and age differ, but they are all continuous. This leads to a number of important implications. Whilst there is general agreement about the identity of, and the appropriate management for, extreme cases, there always remains some scope for disagreement (on grounds of need, efficacy, cost, or balance of risks) about who should be considered a case at all. If only the extremes (e.g. the relatively rare profoundly deaf) were to be viewed as cases, the total numerical and hence resource implications following from slightly changing the definition of a case would be minor. However this is not so, and the resource implications of slightly different definitions can differ greatly. This is true because in adult hearing impairment the area of reasoned disagreement about who might be considered a case falls in a range of severity (20–45 dB HL) where the distribution gives high prevalence. For individuals around the boundary, the implications of where exactly it falls may not be a life-and-death matter. Nevertheless, research on questions of boundary is justified to achieve an evolving definition of candidates for treatment, but this definition has to be sensitive to needs, benefits and costs, if its use is to permit maximum health gain to be realised per unit of resource allocated. Indeed, such a dispassionate cost-utility approach may be easier to introduce where life-and-death matters are **not** involved.

There will be many opportunities for professional and public confusion if terminology, concepts and attitudes appropriate to extreme cases are generalised to marginal cases or *vice versa*. To say in the same sentence that 'deafness' is **both** drastic and prevalent amounts almost to a pun; the impairment level that is the most frequent is not the most drastic and *vice versa*; this follows directly from the prevalence/severity distribution. In the handicap domain this opposition is furthermore a logically necessary truth. A disadvantage can only be scaled as a position relative to other members of society, so the most handicapped are by definition rare.

A part-solution to dilemmas of 'caseness' comes with the terminology of the discipline of audiology, which has long distinguished degrees of impairment via a widely-used category scale of severity. Its six categories are: 'hearing within normal limits', mild, moderate, severe, profound and total hearing loss. Some classificatory schemes insert a seventh 'moderately severe' category in the middle and squeeze the others up the dB HTL scale. The precise physical definitions of the severity scale and of the boundaries between these notional categories need not concern us here. The prevalence/severity distribution is important because gross severity is the most action-relevant item of information about the individual that test data on hearing can so far supply. Chapter 4 quotes prevalences of various severities of impairment in the adult population and describes a method for arriving at the definition of who should be a case. Here, 'case' has to be taken to mean a candidate·for available regimes of management, such as the provision of a hearing aid, rather than providing an instance of a specific disease. The appropriate intervention may be only loosely related to the definition of the disease group. In hearing disorders, the distinction among types of case rests not only largely upon the severity scale for impairment, but also upon other factors, sometimes including the diagnosis of a particular disease. Planning intervention for an individual implies tailoring a package from a range of possibly useful procedures; candidates for intervention are those upon whom it is generally beneficial to expend further efforts, without there necessarily being a set of detailed prescriptions for what each should receive. This leads to a concept of case very close to the definition of a person with a 'need' recently adopted for the UK National Health Service. That definition implies a need for which there exists some effective intervention. As the common term 'needy' means 'indigent', a separate term is required for the individuals with needs; I use the term 'candidate'.

2. EARS OR PEOPLE?

The rhetorical title of this section is not intended to raise any philosophical opposition between holistic and mechanistic medicine. The obvious fact of humans possessing two ears is all too easily over-looked. That oversight leads to mistakes ranging from the inappropriate statistical analysis of data (in which the results for each ear are totalled as if to double the number of cases), through to some patients' refusal to accept two hearing aids, on the grounds that they do not consider themselves sufficiently hard-of-hearing or find one hard enough to cope with. Only the briefest introduction to the psycho-acoustics of binaural hearing is possible here, but some is necessary in order to understand when the focus of investigation should be individual ears, when a pair of ears, and when whole **people**.

In general, the degree of hearing loss on the better-hearing ear is the most important determinant of auditory disability, overriding by a considerable margin most other factors so far examined. This is true whether the further factors examined have reflected other aspects of the pathophysiology of the better ear, factors in the nervous system, or factors in the worse ear. In some circumstances importance also attaches to the worse-hearing ear (or to the asymmetry between the ears for a given better-ear hearing level, which is an alternative way of expressing the same additional information). When the desired signal and undesired noise come from different directions in space, the effective separation of the signal from the noise is greatly helped by the availability of slightly differing information arriving at the two ears. Three types of advantage from the use of the two ears have been distinguished: (i) the greater chance that one particular ear (i.e. either) will be on the side of the signal occurring at a particular moment, and hence have its signal-to-noise ratio improved by the head's acoustic baffle action, which attenuates the high-frequency components of the noise; (ii) statistical summation, helping to overcome the inherent variability in the internal neurophysiological representations of the signal (this improvement occurs even when identical representations of signal plus noise are played to two earphones); (iii) stereophonic hearing, giving, particularly for low-frequency sounds, some differential localisation in space on the basis of slight interaural disparities in time-of-arrival and intensity (which will differ between a signal and a noise separated in space). Averaging over a range of circumstances, these three modes make approximately equal contributions to the advantage of binaural hearing. The possibility of distinguishing three different component bases of binaural advantage that having two ears confers should indicate to the reader the scientific sophistication reached in studies of binaural hearing. This field is particularly mature scientifically because it is relatively easy to experiment comparing one to two ears and because both the stimuli and the processing performed upon them can be described mathematically in ways that are complicated enough to express reality whilst remaining computationally tractable.

A person with only a single functioning ear will be deprived of all of the three beneficial principles of binaural hearing. To describe auditory ability generally, a simplified index emphasising only the role of the better ear is reasonably valid, provided that a generally favourable signal-to-noise ratio can be assumed, for example in dialogue with a single person in quiet, non-reverberant surroundings. Progressive adjustment by the elderly to auditory and other disabilities tends to restrict a significant proportion of their communication to precisely such an acoustical setting, and this may help partly to explain why binaural hearing is sometimes not given the emphasis it deserves. But in noisy environments, one-eared listening is at a grave disadvantage. Given a noisy environment, the 'organ of hearing' is not the ear, but two ears and a brain. This proposition is insufficiently acknowledged in clinical practice and in service provision, and to that extent otology and audiology have been insufficiently holistic.

Asymmetrical hearing ability puts severe stresses upon the mechanisms that enable binaural hearing. Beyond this the detailed implications of asymmetry in hearing disability and in treatment are far-reaching, but have to be acknowledged as being still somewhat unclear. The question arises whether we should count, detect or treat cases with at least one bad ear *versus* cases with two bad ears. This has no simple universal answer. However, in the epidemiology of hearing impairment the issue is of prime importance. With hearing levels on the two ears being likely to diverge in the many cases of unilateral pathology, any decision to take the 'worse' ear into account will bring into scope greater numbers than a criterion based on the better ear alone. Obviously, there will be resource implications.

3. CATEGORIES OF IMPAIRMENT

One more distinction is required for addressing issues in service provision, that between conductive and cochlear hearing impairments. Conductive pathology is located in the middle ear, between the eardrum and the oval window. At this latter point the pressure changes in the air that comprise sound are transferred by movements of the middle ear system of connected bony levers into wave motion in the cochlea; pathology in the middle ear tends to reduce the degree of this transfer. The term 'sensorineural' was introduced in the 1950s as a more satisfactory alternative at the time to 'nerve' or 'perceptive' deafness—as a way to denote non-conductive impairments. In fact the majority of non-conductive hearing disorders are not neural but sensory—sited in the transducer hair cells of the inner ear (cochlea). Due to recent developments in diagnostic imaging, ways of distinguishing neural or retrocochlear disorders from cochlear disorders have progressed greatly; the need for a two-category word, implying some difficulty or undesirability of the distinction between sensory (cochlear) and neural, is disappearing. 'Sensorineural' now has a limited usable life. Even 'sensory' is not a very good term, because it is sometimes also used to describe **all** levels of the sensory system from ear canal to brain, as well as specific transducer functions. The ability to distinguish non-invasively and accurately between sub-sites of pathologies within the cochlea still largely eludes us. It is becoming possible to distinguish faulty hydromechanical transmission of the wave motion from faulty receptor sensitivity to that motion, and it may become possible to distinguish pathology of the inner hair cells from pathology of the outer hair cells although the chances of deriving practical advantage in treatment from this distinction are currently slender.

Conductive hearing loss has long been recognised to be largely attenuative in nature, involving a loss of sensitivity (raised thresholds) and a simple transposition of the dynamic range; as a result amplification is a very adequate solution to the problem. Various non-linear mechanical distortions could also arise within a diseased middle ear, but these appear to be of only secondary importance. Hearing loss due to pathology located in the cochlea involves various forms of analyser of degradation in addition to the basic loss of threshold sensitivity. The main two are: (a) loss of dynamic range, i.e. an uncomfortable loudness level very little (if at all) raised from normal, thus restricting the scope for amplification; and (b) loss of frequency resolution (hence the noise-proneness in cochlear impairments associated with age, introduced in Chapter 1). This simple distinction between conductive and cochlear hearing loss has stood the test of time extraordinarily well, but a number of factors make it less hard-and-fast that textbooks imply:

(i) Compound pathology. Many pathological processes can spread or cause secondary pathology via space occupation, restriction of blood supply, microbial or enzymatic penetration, etc. Mostly, the implications concern slightly raised risk of cochlear pathology in diseases of the middle ear such as otosclerosis and chronic suppurative otitis media in adults, and to a lesser extent in secretory otitis media in children. Such 'mixed' losses are fairly common and comprise a high proportion of severe hearing losses.

(ii) Level-dependence. In general, conductive forms of hearing disorder are correctly viewed as ultimately 'less serious' than cochlear or neural forms, because the analyser is not damaged; loud speech, reconstructive surgery of the middle ear and hearing aids can all be highly effective. However, under many of the circumstances causing common, if minor difficultes, the reverse may be true. Unless intensity levels above those of conversational speech can be arranged (by shouting, high amplifier volume settings, etc.) the person with the typical mild-to-moderate conductive hearing impairment of middle-ear origin is actually worse off than the person with a nominally equivalent cochlear loss of sensitivity.

(iii) Central deprivation effects. The central nervous system modifies its response in many ways to transformations in its sensory inputs. This is especially true during early development, at which stage severe sensory deprivation may permanently compromise maturation of the central processes that mediate discrimination, indentification and recognition of sounds such as speech. The evidence is considered in more detail in the following chapter. For the present, it is sufficient to observe that a long-term conductive loss (even a moderate one, because of point (ii) above) may lead to types of abnormality other than the original loss of peripheral sensitivity. Such developmental deficits may require rather sophisticated assessment to distinguish their indirect effects from effects arising directly through pathology in the cochlea.

REFERENCES

1. FREELAND, A. P., (1989). *Deafness: the facts*. Oxford University Press.
2. KATZ, J., (Ed) (1985). *Handbook of Clinical Audiology*. WILLIAMS & WILLIAMS: Baltimore.

3

HEARING IMPAIRMENTS IN CHILDREN

PRE-LINGUAL HEARING IMPAIRMENT PROVIDES A WIDELY ACCEPTED instance of secondary prevention, in turn justifying the prime instance of universal (mass) screening for hearing problems. In this chapter, I examine two rather different aspects of the problem of case-finding in childhood. I draw heavily on the work of my colleagues Adrian Davis and Mark Lutman on the detection of congenital cochlear impairment, and on my own critical review of research in public health aspects of screening for hearing impairment and in the epidemiology of otitis media. Much of the latter is available in an HMSO report co-authored with Eamonn Hughes[1] for the Department of Health, or else has been stimulated by doing that review. Congenital cochlear impairments of hearing contrast markedly with otitis media in terms of prevalence, severity, timing and form of intervention (Table 3.1). However I discuss the two conditions in the same chapter to illustrate their mutual impact in service terms, and to draw on common evidence and arguments for early detection.

1. EARLY DETECTION OF PRE-LINGUAL COCHLEAR HEARING IMPAIRMENT

Children born with hearing impairment around 1960 preceded both the widespread introduction of mass screening for hearing impairment, and the general spread of awareness among health service professions and the public at large of the adverse consequences of early auditory deprivation. The same children, on leaving schools for the deaf and units for the partially hearing in the mid 1970s were documented[2] as having immense verbal and cognitive deficits, that were not explicable by any associated

References begin on p. 79.

TABLE 3.1 *The two main forms of hearing impairment in childhood*

	Pre-lingual Cochlear Impairment	Otitis media with effusion (OME)
Main Pathology	Unformed or damaged transducer cells	Viscous fluid in middle ear
Severity range	20–120 dBHTL	0–50 dBHTL
Nominal Prevalence	Under 1:1000 at 50 dBHTL (better ear)	(Point prevalence) 15–25% lower in summer persistent histories about 5%
Shape of distribution of prevalence by: (a) Severity (b) Persistence	(a) Roughly flat (b) Permanent	(a) Symmetrical about 25 dBHTL (b) Exponential tail
Timing	Life-long from birth or early childhood	Prevalence plateau about 9 months–6 years
Interventions	From about 30 dBHTL to about 105 dBHTL hearing aids (usually binaural) thought essential in language learning period and usually thereafter Degree of benefit somewhat limited in 30–40 and 90–105 dB range	Surgery effective in improving hearing levels if above about 25 dBHTL for 6–9 months Hearing aids potentially effective, but rarely used, due to problem coping in some families

pathology of the central nervous system. The size of these deficits is suggested by the reading age of eight years, contrasting with the expected 16 years or thereabouts. Such evidence has been interpreted by some as a failure of 'oral' education, i.e. as a failure of 'misguided' attempts to treat such children as 'non-deaf', by forcing unachievable goals of speaking and aural understanding upon them, by denying them the use of signing, or all of these. The criticism was, in part, valid, and there is every reason to make signing available to children who are established early as having no useful sound input, and also to other children likely to suffer severe communication disability. However, a more far-reaching interpretation of the findings invokes the early plasticity of the nervous system,[3] and the necessity of early auditory input to enable language learning, and thence to allow the full development of a differentiated cognitive system of verbal skills and social concepts.

Early detection of children with severe hearing impairments began to occur in significant numbers after about 1970. Teachers working with deaf children observed some early-aided children attaining higher levels of linguistic performance than formerly thought possible. To know how general the improvement has been, a formal study of levels of educational achievement is now needed, with the earlier data on reading and other tests as historical controls. This would need to take some account of shift in aetiologies (e.g. reduced rubella incidence) and to document the actual ages of initial use of hearing aids. Recent evidence, looking at age-of-detection within samples of hearing-impaired children[4,5] argues for a beneficial effect of the early detection in severe and profound pre-lingual impairment. There are great difficulties in obtaining extensive evidence in the most controlled form that would enable this benefit from early aiding to be asserted without reservation. Firstly, the number of affected children in any one district is small, giving problems of sample sizes. Secondly, the outcome for a particular child depends upon other factors in the individual child and in the family. Thirdly, a controlled trial is impossible; withholding awareness from parents and withholding treatment (i.e. not providing hearing aids nor (re)habilitation of communication skills to the evidently impaired children) would generally not be ethical. This ethical objection would stand against withholding rehabilitation as tertiary prevention from a population. Some practitioners could perhaps be convinced to provide a control group, on the basis that doubt remained in respect of any major **additional** benefit from specifically early provision to achieve secondary prevention. Fourthly, the naturally occurring variation in age at detection reflects aspects of the family that are likely also to have major effects on eventual communication skills—for example, its health awareness and its emphasis upon oral communication. Thus, except where the unbiased effect of a screen has been responsible, early-detected children are probably also luckier in other ways. Finally, it is difficult to ensure the full effective and consistent use of hearing aids by the family and child, so potential benefits are not realised in every instance, introducing some variability.

The argument for early identification has relied in part on the generalisation of evidence from sensory deprivation experiments in animals[3] and the associated hypothesis of 'critical' (sensitive) periods in the stimulated development of the central nervous system. That evidence gives some grounds for the belief that early auditory experience is important, and that not all of the deficit due to deprivation can be made up. Another piece of evidence is the pattern seen in children who become profoundly hearing-impaired later in childhood. Although the stress and interpersonal adjustment problems can be even greater in these children, the deficit in communication and conceptualisation seems not to be so marked. These post-lingually affected children, typically with progressive conditions, head injury, mumps or meningitis, comprise under 20 per cent of the target group and usually indicate or display signs of their deafness fairly soon. In most contexts it is therefore mistaken to cite the non-congenital cases as justification for mass screening after early childhood. Despite these loose ends, the argument for early intervention has not been cogently questioned, perhaps partially explaining why the difficulties in acquiring more extensive and direct evidence for it have not had to be faced so far. Attitudes and experiences of parents have also played a powerful role in not questioning the orthodoxy; in systems for child health surveillance that lack highly effective early screens (i.e. in most such systems), parents of severely deaf children have often had battles to convince medical personnel that something was wrong with their child. The converse instances, where parents have been surprised by professional detection of hearing impairment, are even more numerous, although they do not of course figure so dramatically in personal narratives. After both types of oversight, parents tend to claim in retrospect that they would rather have known earlier, or are glad that the knowledge came no later. To be fair, denial by parents of their own suspicions can also occur, where they cannot face coping with the implications.

I am more concerned here to fine-tune the orthodox argument for early detection, than to question it outright. The consensus has been widely accepted in a public health context[6,7] that pre-lingual impairment needs to be found early by some sort of screening process. This acceptance has played down the need to obtain evidence of the highest scientific quality favouring the critical period hypothesis. However demands for demonstrations of efficacy have now become important in the competition for resources. In this context the extent, control and quantitative sophistication of the evidence published to date is sufficient to justify further research to demonstrate benefit for early intervention. The priority for more widespread routine implementation of very early screening has to depend on the strength of that evidence of benefit. The nature of the evidence required will shift with changes in patterns of health care and with the aetiological profile of children having severe and profound hearing losses, so conclusions on the effects of early aiding would need to be reviewed every 10–15 years and new evidence supplied. Ramkalawan and Davis[5] assembled a sample of severely/profoundly deaf children without other handicaps to investigate the effect of age at which a hearing aid had been provided. While arguments for early aiding apply equally to the multi-handicapped, the restriction is important methodologically, partly for securing a clearer result. The improvements in early detection rates in recent years in the district covered meant that there were sufficient numbers of children provided with aids before 18 months of age. They found (after extracting the obvious effect of age at time of test) significant beneficial effects of early aiding on simple metrics of emerging language and communication.

In children it is not certain over what range of hearing impairments the early intervention argument applies for screening as a step to secondary prevention. Current hearing aids give little benefit when fitted to ears of adults with hearing losses less than about 25–30 dB HTL, and the quality of technology (and hence the costs) have to be high to avoid providing an aid which is only an expensive and noisy earplug! A loss of 35–40 dB is a more typical boundary beyond which benefit, though variable, is broadly assured. Does the appropriate qualifying hearing level occur at a similar value in children? If so, there may be a limit or criterion on the severity at which it is worth aiming a screen. The extra needs of the children learning a language could justify aiding at milder levels overall than in adults, provided that effective fitting and use of aids of good quality can be guaranteed. However, difficulties of ensuring in a young child the appropriate choice of optimum aid characteristics and stimulation levels, and of verifying proper functioning and use of the aid argue more cautiously. Given these difficulties, it is arguable that the margin of advantage occurs around similar levels of impairment in children and adults. This dilemma refers to cochlear impairments; as we have seen,[8] different arguments will apply in conductive impairment. For cochlear impairment it has been argued[9] that any boundary which reflects the absolute degree of need will have to depend upon whether the child also has other problems, i.e. is multi-handicapped. The multi-handicapped group overlaps considerably with the group that passes through neonatal intensive care, so in practice this point amounts to justifying a somewhat milder screening level or referral criterion for such an at-risk group than might be justified in the general population. Taken together, these considerations balance out, leaving no overriding audiological reason to separate the audiometric criterion for candidature for hearing aids in children from that in adults, insofar as individual ears are concerned.

Unfortunately, it is generally difficult to derive firm evidence to substantiate guidelines from the available literature concerning which children should receive an aid. Many factors other than the aidability of individual ears determine the benefit from and the continued use of hearing aids, not least the somewhat variable extent to which they have been appropriately set and maintained in good working order. So far, the absence of precise criteria for aiding has in practice not been a great obstacle to specifying screening targets, because provision of a hearing aid will not be unambiguously recommended in every instance. The consequences of detection for parental awareness and compensatory communicative behaviour are probably more beneficial than they may be anxiety-provoking, stigmatising or dependency-inducing. This statement applies down to the minimum level that can be detected in screening. This level lies at about 25-30 dB HTL, but the precise level depends on the particular technology used and on the relative acceptability of screening errors of the false-positive versus the false-negative type. The problem of candidature for hearing aids and targeting of screens is examined in more detail in Section 4 of this Chapter.

TABLE 3.2 *Fourteen principles of screening*

The first ten principles were proposed by Wilson and Jungner (Reference 10) and the remaining four by Haggard (Reference 11). The complete set was adopted by the Medical Research Council's Health Services and Public Health Research Board as principles to guide research in which an actual screening programme was to be implemented, and principles 13 and 14 are particularly relevant to research and development. Principle 14 is required because many screens find more than one type of case.

1. The condition screened for should be an important health problem.

2. There should be an accepted treatment for cases identified.

3. Facilities for diagnosis and treatment should be available.

4. There should be a recognisable latent or early symptomatic stage.

5. There should be a suitable test or examination.

6. The test should be acceptable to the population.

7. The natural history of the condition should be understood.

8. There should be an agreed policy on whom to treat as patients.

9. The cost of case-finding (including diagnosis and treatment of patients diagnosed) should be non-wastefully balanced in relation to expenditure or medical care as a whole.

10. Case-finding should be a continuing process and not 'once and for all'.

11. The incidental harm done by the screening, and by the information (correct or otherwise) that it gives should be small in relation to the benefits from the screening-assessment-treatment system.

12. There should be agreed guidelines on whom, when and how to tell the provisional and the final results, and there should be transitional counselling support.

13. All screening arrangements should be reviewed from time to time in the light of changes in demography, culture, health services, and the epidemiology of the target conditions.

14. Costs and effectiveness, plus the benefits of screening and the consequential assessments and treatments, have to be considered on a stratified e.g. (demographic or case-type) basis, and their effectiveness and benefit maximised in each stratum.

2. DECISIONS TO INTRODUCE OR CHANGE SCREENS

In determining whether or not a screen should exist, some 14 principles need to be satisfied (Table 3.2). These are the classical ten of Wilson and Jungner[10] plus four of my own.[11] Principles 1, 2, 4 and 8 are abstract statements of the issues introduced concretely in the preceding 2 paragraphs. Principles 2 and 3 in essence oblige the advocate of routine screening to have already produced evidence of material health gain and of having reliable arrangements for diagnosis and treatment to follow up the screening. Demonstrating the technological virtuosity in detecting asymptomatic disease or future disability is only a first research step. It is not a sufficient basis for introducing mass screening. Even **research** on techniques would be unethical without some form of service for cases identified; obviously, until enough early cases have been located to specify a treatment, outline the service and do the appropriate intervention trials, that service may have to be rudimentary. Principle 4, with its emphasis on progression seems to require a demonstration of secondary rather than merely tertiary prevention. I do not regard this principle as overriding; it is not a logical or ethical requirement for screening, that the target condition would necessarily deteriorate or be compounded if left undetected for a longer time. However, if only tertiary prevention is assured, the magnitude of the health gain and the extent to which the other principles of screening are met should be closely examined before implementing a screen. This point is made to illustrate that the principles of screening should not be invoked over-rigidly, nor in isolation.

Audiology offers some instances of public health gain derived from screens that do not display total conformity to the 14 principles. As an example, about one sixth of the population of the UK lives in districts which now have some form of neonatal at-risk screening programme, even if the coverage of children at risk in these districts is not complete. A paediatric audiology service is **in theory** available at a level acceptable for this population, as are free hearing aids. However, in practice it is far from clear that the necessary skill levels and staff time are available everywhere for precise diagnostic measurement of hearing in babies a few days or weeks olds. The appropriate levels of skill for properly fitting and adjusting appropriate hearing aids for (re)habilitating the very youngest children are certainly not available to the corresponding population. In line with principle 3, the rate at which neonatal screening—even on an at-risk basis—can spread would be limited by the rate at which paediatric audiology services more generally can be brought up to scratch. For this reason a recent set of recommendations on screening[1] had also to include a recommendation to improve these services.

Most health districts in the UK still have a two-part system for screening children's hearing. Firstly, there is the behavioural screen of hearing by the distraction test administered at between 7 and 9 months by health visitors, virtually ubiquitous since about 1970. When the test is properly implemented[12] the baby is held on the parent's knee and an accomplice distracts the baby's attention with visible activity and sound onto a low table in front e.g. with a toy such as a small spinning top. The toy is stilled and hidden by the accomplice's hand. The baby's attention does not wander for an interval of a few seconds, and during this interval standard sounds are presented at one or other side at a standard distance and out of view. Response is measured by a head turn; criteria for a genuine turn have to be met within a specified interval. More intense auditory clues such as footfalls or creaks, and visual clues such as shadows or eye-contact have to be rigorously precluded, or a child may wrongly 'pass'. The number of stimulus presentations is specified, as are referral criteria (generally a second non-response on re-test after one month, if the child 'fails' or is untestable).

In good screening implementations, the modified distraction test can have high sensitivity.[9] In the hands of skilled clinical personnel, it can be an excellent test for 6- to 11-month old children, suitable for assessment of frequency-specific hearing levels, as required in the fitting of hearing aids. However, clinical professional groups are not generally educated to exercise precise physical control over stimuli and behavioural testing procedures. One of the eight meanings of the word 'clinical' is 'informal'. Criticisms have abounded of the poorly implemented testing procedures with non-specialising screeners and of the misapplied referral rules, that jointly comprise the typical screen. Behavioural skills and specific training in technique are required in at least one, but preferably two, testers, so that the cautions listed above can be observed. This, plus the need for an accomplice, and for an ordinarily quiet acoustical environment, make it evident that cost and effectiveness in the typical implementation by health visitors are going to be problematic. This is not to deny that excellent implementations of screening with the distraction test do exist[12] and achieve many early detections. Nevertheless, it is not clear that the political will can be found to commandeer the resources needed to overcome the problems of implementation and scarce skills. Screening with the distraction test has to be considered as a medium-term stop-gap, as this test lacks the fool-proof simplicity and robustness required of a test suited to mass screening. A number of authorities are discontinuing it on the basis of the short-comings of implementation in their own districts. However this is by no means a straightforward course, as the issue of a suitable arrangement to replace universal screening by be-havioural test is not settled. Giving awareness and responsibility to parents may be culturally admirable and of low cost, but it does not produce highly effective results; perhaps one in five deaf children at most can be detected by parents alerted to be suspi-cious of hearing impairment in their children.[13] With minor modifications, the distraction test has been used clinically for over 50 years and used in screening for about 25. It may be some time before any more cost-effective overall system covering the not-at-risk can be put in place, but when that time comes the retirement can be honourable. Consideration of what the replacement might be requires an impartial assessment of the system for child health surveillance as a whole. Single-tester behavioural tests of hear-ing—if shown to be reliable and valid—may have some role to play. The effectiveness is most unlikely to be higher, but the cost would be lower.

The second standard form of provisions is currently the screen at school entry, which in many of the old local authorities already existed in the 1930s as part of the school medical services, and which became nearly ubiquitous in the 1950s. This usually in-volves a 'sweep' i.e. pure-tone stimuli of standard frequencies at screening levels of 20 or 25 dB, followed by full threshold determi-nation if any tone is not heard. The main short-term yield from this screen is large numbers of cases happening to have fluid in their ears on the test day, of whom a proportion will have persis-tent histories of otitis media. The numbers of pre-lingually cochlear-impaired children still undetected by school age ought to be extremely small, if the rest of the child health surveillance system is working well; however, there are several other reasons for keeping this screen, and very few districts have abandoned it.

The two standard screens are supplemented by a variety of surveillance arrangements in the intervening years.

Changes to the total system could involve reducing or increasing the number of screening occasions, and/or changing their nature and timing. So, for example, if an effective neonatal screen were to come into force and the 7–9 month distraction test screen were subsequently to be abandoned, it could then be argued that resources spent on screening at school could be better spent at the pre-school stage to avoid the gap of nearly five years with no screening test. This might justify the development of an appropriately standardised test for $2\frac{1}{2}$–$3\frac{1}{2}$ year olds. About one third of health authorities do have a notionally universal screen at $2\frac{1}{2}$–$3\frac{1}{2}$ years involving some non-standardised behavioural test of hearing. Such arrangements can readily be criticised on multiple grounds.[1] Not merely is practice diverse, with aims unclear and no monitoring data published on the yield, but the epidemiological case for even starting the development work on a screening test with appropriate properties for the age range has never been coherently stated. In particular, strict limits to the possible yield are set by the low coverage (50–80 per cent by the age of three) generally achievable in a supposedly universal screen, taken together with the 'inverse care law'. This law states that the individuals or strata in society most needing services tend least to receive them. A special instance of the inverse care law is the tendency for people who do not keep screening appointments for a variety of reasons, to come from population strata more likely to experience the condition screened for.[14] A more promising use of resources than incomplete screening of $2\frac{1}{2}$–$3\frac{1}{2}$ year olds might be to target that minority **not** having attended other screening appointments, or to define some risk basis whereby a group highly at risk could be defined, and where the extra effort needed to ensure high coverage would become justified.

Choosing the best ages for a set of screens is complex, because in any viable screen three crucial factors depend upon age: the appropriate class of test method, the numbers with the target condition (still) present in the population at the age in question, and the receptiveness of the population to preventive health measure such as screening. A fourth consideration is also important in practice—the linkage to other aspects of child health surveillance. Regrettably, advocates of a particular solution often concentrate

upon one of these factors, or perhaps two. Some further epidemiology is necessary to fully appreciate why all are relevant.

In the discussion so far I have already avoided use of the usual
terms 'sensitivity' and 'specificity' as applied to screening. These
two measures (or equivalent transformations of them) provide an
appropriate way of expressing the accuracy of a screening test
(against a more definitive diagnostic test) plus the location of the
decision criterion or bias towards negative (passing) *versus* positive
(failing). These indices are of concern both to researchers developing tests and to personnel deciding on the implementation of
cost-effective screening systems. The properties of the test which
they reflect do impose limits on screen performance, but other
factors may have more bearing upon the real utility of a screen—
factors such as **coverage** and **incremental yield**, both of which
influence the sensitivity that is achievable in practice. Coverage is
the proportion of the target population that actually receives the
screening test. Whether the target group is all children (universal)
or some at-risk sub-population, ideally 100 per cent of the
specified target group should receive the test. This is never fully
achievable, but the inverse care law makes very high coverage a
necessity, which in turn has implications for cost. It will now be
seen why purporting to quote the 'sensitivity' of a screen in routine
services can be misleading, over and above the usual difficulty of
being sure that all false-negative cases have eventually been documented, which a true sensitivity index pre-supposes. A **test** with
very high sensitivity that is used in a **screen** of low coverage will
still produce a low yield. The term 'sensitivity of a **screen**' can
thus be ambiguous, and is even misleading if it is the (more
favourable) **test** sensitivity that is quoted. Typical achievable coverage for reasons of administrative feasibility or attendance at
screening appointments drops from about 99 per cent at maternity for at-risk intensive care children, to 85–98 per cent at 9
months and to 50–80 per cent at three years, depending upon the
population and the resources devoted to pursuit.[1] It then rises to
about 99 per cent at school entry. The choice of the setting for
implementation—preferably a captive population—is therefore as
important as the choice of test. Incremental yield is simply the
number or proportion of cases not found by any other means
before the age in question.

The concepts of incremental yield and coverage bring us directly to the problem of planning an optimum set of sequentially dependent screens to cover childhood. Quoting the incremental yield of a screen also de-emphasises the sensitivity of a test to abnormalities generally, and emphasises instead the number of hitherto undetected cases that the screen will in practice find. Put simply, a child found early is no longer in the pool to be found, so any early screen reduces the yield from any later screen, possibly threatening its viability. The concrete dimensions of this problem are sketched in Figure 3.1.

3. NEONATAL SCREENING

Neonatal screening is making progress on an at-risk basis, with up to one fifth of health districts in the UK already having or planning some provision. It has already been amply demonstrated that such screens are feasible and that they do find hearing-impaired babies but a decision on widespread implementation of at-risk neonatal screening is still a little way off, and one on universal screening at this age not due for some years. Current research is optimising the testing technology, establishing screen performance, and monitoring the reliability of implementation. The neonatally at-risk (for reasons of low birth weight, perinatal trauma, or infection) already require and receive a high level of medical care for a prolonged period, and they are accessible because captive for several days. The numbers in the other main group identifiable as at risk, those with a family history of pre-lingual deafness, are small, but their level of risk is highly raised; this justifies administrative resources in pursuit of this target group also. Unfortunately the sensitivity of practicable questions for parents about the relevant type of family history is poor, so implementation is not straightforward, and may have to vary according to the way that local services in both health and social support are organised. The conjunction of these groups makes it possible to realise the potential advantage of finding almost 50 per cent of all hearing-impaired babies by testing only about 7 per cent of all babies. Babies with craniofacial abnormalities may also be routed into the screen, but as they would mostly be referred for full audiological assessment, this provision should not be seen as a source of major improvement.

My emphasis in this account of the very early detection of hearing impairment deliberately avoids the widespread misunder-

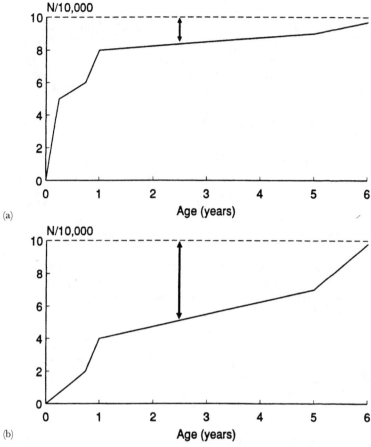

(a)

(b)

FIGURE 3.1 A conceptual diagram to illustrate the concept of actual incremental yield. The actual incremental yield is the product of the number of cases still remaining, with the coverage of the screen and the sensitivity of the test. The reference population is assumed to have an annual birth cohort of 10,000 and to produce eventually 10 cases at 50dB HTL better ear. There is assumed to be a continuous trickle of detections not arising in the preventive screening system. The number of hearing-impaired children remaining at any stage to be detected depends on the cohort prevalence, on the incidence of post-natally acquired cases, and on the success of previous attempts to detect cases. The first panel (a) assumes an effective neonatal at-risk system with 50% of cases (5 per 10,000) found post-natally. The second step in the function represents a screen at 8 months with a test that is only 50% sensitive. This raises the issue of whether such a screen could be cost-effective and especially whether one occurring later (arrows) can be effective. In panel (b), with no neonatal screen, and an ineffective 8-month screen (2/8 = 25% sensitivity), there might well be some point in a later screen or surveillance arrangement from the point of view of incremental yield of a single screen. From the point of view of the system as a whole, this would be an admission of defeat.

standing that screening gadgets can suddenly emerge that on their own 'solve' problems of screening. If only the matter were so simple! Challenging though the bio-engineering problems are, they are over-shadowed by the public health problems. All high technology requires an informed user and a monitoring process involving skilled and knowledgeable personnel. After some preliminary experimentation with behavioural technology for testing neonates that turned out to be under-specific and only sensitive to the severest impairments,[15] two serious contender technologies are now available. The first is an abbreviated and semi-automated form of a more elaborate diagnostic test—the coherently averaged electrical brainstem response (ABR) evoked at the scalp by repeated auditory stimuli, usually clicks.[16] The second is the evoked oto-acoustic emission (EOAE). This reflects a non-linear active mechanical response in the cochlea[17] which I deliberately omitted from the introduction to hearing science in Chapter 2. In brief, the outer hair cells act as a local amplifier for frequency-selective movements of the cochlear partition. This active non-linear process is evident in the intermodulation distortion products to continuous combinations of tones (DPOAE), and in the 'echoes' to repeated click transients (CEOAE).[18] In terms of the simplicity, non-invasiveness and robustness required in screening applications, neither ABR nor EOAE is totally ideal. EOAE has the edge for an initial test in being slightly less invasive and requiring a much shorter test time (about 5–10 as opposed to 30–40 min per child). It nevertheless requires a quiescent baby, careful regular calibration, careful placement of the probe in the ear and a non-trivial level of understanding, organisation and skill on the part of the screener. Current implementations of CEOAE furthermore require a quiet room.

Sensitivity of both the ABR and EOAE technique is high enough (95–99 per cent to constitute no obstacle to application. Specificity is an obstacle, particularly for EOAEs, as they often do not produce a response at birth. This is due either to some aspect of maturation not yet understood or to the fact that many newborns in the at-risk group have fluid-filled ears for a few days, which this technique also detects, although this is not what is ultimately of concern. The amplitude of the CEOAE does not grow in proportion to the amplitude of stimulation; this non-linear property makes it a somewhat all-or-none phenomenon, ideal for screening. Unfortunately the non-linearity does not allow repeat testing at a raised level corresponding to the expected effect of presence of fluid; even if an emission is triggered in the middle ear it cannot propagate out through the fluid. In contrast, ABR allows a hearing level to be obtained and any conductive hearing loss to be discounted from the pattern of results obtained by re-testing at different intensities. This is half way to a diagnostic rather than a screening test, but a necessary accompaniment due is the high prevalence of fluid in the ear in newborn children. With such tests as ABR the stimulus level can be varied at will, also allowing some choice intensity of referral criterion. One suggestion for overcoming the all-or-none problem with EOAE is to use the ABR at a raised stimulation level to immediately sift through those failing the EOAE test; this has been shown[19] to reduce to acceptable proportions the referral rates to full assessment, and hence the costs and the parental anxieties. An advantage in this combination is that differing referral criteria from the ABR stage could be used in different risk groups, e.g. a lower criterion for the perinatally at-risk than for either a family history or the not-at-risk children in universal screening. However, whether differing criteria would be widely applied in this way is uncertain, as the essence of screening is simplicity and standardisation. There is an understandable professional reluctance to inhibit the referral of any child coming under suspicion, whatever the uncertainty of this suspicion or the probable mildness of the condition. The capital cost of having two types of equipment available would only be a small part of the cost of such a method, the professional and administrative time being the major one. Precise costs are currently being documented for this dual-test screening, but appear to be under £5,000 per case detected in at-risk (targeted) neonatal screening. For universal screening they would be much higher.

As technology progresses, much of its economic benefit lies in its spread through increased volume at lower cost of production. Part of this diffusion process depends on increased sophistication to increase its utility in the hands of people of minimum training. The expectation of diffusion justifies not only research towards achieving the ideal metric properties of a test for screening applications, but also attention to the ergonomics of its widespread use, so as to achieve the anticipated cost reductions. Experience with the two techniques suitable for neonatal screening has demonstrated implementation difficulties in creating and maintaining the necessary skill, understanding and motivation when staff of low professional grading are used, even when given training in the procedure. It remains unproven for the ABR and EAOE technologies whether or not routine results of adequate quality can be obtained with staff at the level of basic nursing qualifications or less. Hence very precise costings would be premature; an upper-bound cost element for an appropriate staffing grade should therefore be used in quoted costings until this question is settled. More generally, factors such as the number of maternity sites serving a given district population will also bear upon the logistics and costs and prohibit the quoting of a single definitive cost per child detected. Research currently in progress is attempting to define the efficiency and cost of various alternative technologies and systems. It seems likely that one of the physiological techniques, or the dual combination mentioned, will indeed turn out to be cost-effective, in comparison with typical implementations of screens based on the distraction test at 7–9 months. This comparison is likely to be favourable to at-risk neonatal screening in terms of cost per child detected, even before counting the probable additional benefit from earlier detection in the individual. For **universal** neonatal screening *versus* a 7–9 month screen with the distraction test, the comparison on cost will be closer and cannot yet reliably be done. Certainly, even with at-risk neonatal screening, the detection of up to one half of the target cases before one month of age does wonders for the main performance indicator of the screening system, namely the distribution of ages at detection.

Neonatal screening on an at-risk basis brings in the wake of its singular efficiency a source of intellectual dissatisfaction, particularly for the egalitarian—the fact that half the target cases are not catered for at all. Callous though this may seem, we have in the limit to accept, in principle, that some groups cannot realistically be included in preventive health arrangements on the grounds of disproportionate cost in locating them; low coverage through consistent inattendance could provide an example, where this is known to be due to intransigence rather than to administrative failure. However for a not-at-risk group, one half of all cases is much too high a percentage to relinquish without serious exploration of viable alternative arrangements. An appropriate means of case-finding among children not readily established as at raised risk is required, along with a rigorous analysis of which types of comparative trial will now be most informative. Figure 3.1 shows that the potential incremental yield is small after any first screen that is worth having, and that there is also a substantial background rate of detection from the reactive process involving parents and general practitioners in 'negotiated referral'. Even though parents can contribute only about a further one fifth of cases, the numbers remaining after the processes (i.e. the actual incremental yield) become small, and the size of any trial to demonstrate any advantage of particular supplementary arrangements has therefore to become very large.

If neonatal screening on an at-risk basis completes its current post-implementation trials successfully and is implemented in most districts, competition will then occur among various proposals as to how a system comprising both neonatal at-risk screening and universal school-entry screening can be supplemented in the most cost-effective way. One of, or some combination of, the following five chief possibilities might be appropriate: (a) universal neonatal screening, (b) an improved screen at 7–9 months based in the immediate future upon the distraction test, (c) surveillance arrangements at various ages (if specifiable and susceptible to monitoring), (d) a risk-based selective screen by some appropriate test between $2\frac{1}{2}$ and $3\frac{1}{2}$ years, or (d) a universal screen around this age. These alternatives are highly disparate in context and target age, and would involve very different techniques. The cases remaining to be detected after these various possibilities would differ between the alternatives in form, severity, age of onset and permanence. The costing of the corresponding services is not simple, and the comparison of benefits would be problematic, due to the difficulty of scaling the benefit from early intervention. One could impose some arbitrary scaling of the time axis (such as logarithmic) in order to condense the effect of later years and so weight an early detection more highly as to benefit. However, the system eventually to be favoured would have to be well ahead of the others for its advantage to be robust across different scaling assumptions. If the differences between systems are small, the calculated advantage for each can depend heavily upon the nature of these assumptions; thus it is necessary to examine the effect of varying the assumptions.

The list of difficulties raised and the various ways of combining elements into a total screening system suggest a long research agenda. As a start, advocates historically committed to, or currently favouring, one or other of the possible screens to supplement neonatal at risk screening need to admit the great uncertainty about costs and benefits, and to see the fallacy of considering one screen in isolation. Proposals must be judged as implementable before the searchlight of data-gathering is turned upon them. For example, proponents of universal neonatal screening must say how a system could guarantee 98–99 per cent coverage on the basis of typical maternity stays of only about 24 hours. Emphasising the importance of coverage may seem to be stating the obvious; however, it is remarkable how accounts of the past or proposals for the future can overlook it. The five-way choice is difficult to address in research because of the large populations required in research on conditions of low prevalence. For congenital pre-lingual healthy cases, current fertility rates would require a project to be either long-term and retrospective, or else to tap a population base of two million to examine each system of screening proposed. This could need at least three English health regions (i.e. populations of several millions) to agree to standardise their implementation of the common elements in the total system (e.g. neonatal at-risk screen as background plus school-entry as follow-up screen through all their districts). Two regions would then need to implement differing but uniform supplementary elements—for example the two most promising from the above list of five—while the third acted as control without these supplementary elements.

4. DECISIONS TO IMPLEMENT

The foregoing analysis has deliberately deferred the detailed but ultimately important question of precisely which children are the target of screening systems, and whether the target should vary with age or circumstances. Several ascertainment studies, particularly those on populations receiving ineffective surveillance and hence reliant on reactive mechanisms, show a natural tendency for severe deficits to be referred earliest and for milder ones to emerge only later.[1] This arises because a more severe impairment will more rapidly become symptomatic in terms of behavioural consequences—usually language delay in the instance of hearing impairment. Taken over a time scale of five years rather than one year, this tendency leads to a general paradox seen in child health surveillance: if the screening test is sensitive to mild impairments, screening will make a **large** difference to the age of detection in the **milder** cases (less able to achieve very high benefit, having less absolute need). However, it may make only a **modest** difference to the detection rate of detection age of more **severe** cases (those more able to benefit, and having greater absolute need). The argument for screening has therefore to rely partly on the benefits of advancement of detection by a year or so in the severe cases, partly on an advancement of 2–4 years in milder cases. Thus, arriving at even a rather general and qualitative estimate of the comparative benefits from various screening systems requires consideration of the numbers to be found at each severity, i.e. consideration of the prevalence-severity distribution.

The prevalence of congenital severe/profound hearing impairment can only be established economically from service-based records; it is too low to document both accurately and cost-effectively in a population study. Amongst the milder cases of those conventionally thought to need audiological help, under-counting cannot entirely be ruled out, as the imperatives towards seeking help are insufficient to guarantee consultation and the uptake of continuing care. Mild cases may be known to one care agency but not to all. It appears that the prevalence-severity distribution for pre-lingual permanent hearing impairment is rather flat (Table 3.3) unlike the distribution with the typical dwindling tail of severe cases found in adults. For many years a figure of 'one child per thousand born deaf' has been quoted. A study by Davis and Wood[9] provides an unbiased statistical account of pre-lingual impairment. It post-dates the reduction in rubella as a major aetiology, and reflects contemporary patterns of survival of children of low birth weight and other perinatal problems. Their sample was constructed from service records, the chief entry criterion being fitting for hearing aids; the large district sampled has good audiology services and a preventive orientation. However, it was not a prospective study of a population cohort, so may be assumed to have slightly under-ascertained in the mild impairment zone, (i.e. at HTL values less than about 40 dB, the limit down to which, for a child, benefit from hearing aids appears to be fairly certain). More than 1:1000 children apparently need

TABLE 3.3 *Prevalence of sensorineural/mixed congenital or progressive hearing impairments*

Severity of hearing impairment (dB HTL)	Overall	Non-NICU	NICU
< 50	0·29	0·20	1·70
50 +	1·06	0·78	5·80
65 +	0·74	0·51	4·60
80 +	0·48	0·37	2·30
95 +	0·29	0·24	1·15
50–64	0·32	0·27	1·15
65–79	0·26	0·14	2·20
80–94	0·19	0·14	1·15
95 +	0·29	0·24	1·15

The prevalences per 1000 births (from Davis and Wood, Reference 9) were obtained in an intensive study of a district with good screening and audiology services plus an intensive care unit. The district has a wide catchment from which inflow cases were excluded, so as to minimise biases. The middle field gives the cumulative distributions, the lower field the banded distributions. 'NICU' denotes those children who graduated from neonatal intensive care, in whom impairments are 8·5 times (1·7/0·2) as prevalent. If those with a family history or orofacial abnormalities are transferred from the non-NICU group into the risk group, the relative risk approaches 15, making at-risk neonatal screening highly advantageous compared to universal neonatal screening. Although the modest sample size shows some fluctuations in prevalence from a band to band, it is evident from the only shallow vertical trend in the lower field that the prevalence/severity distribution is essentially flat, not the exponential tail that would be expected with a normal distribution of severity.

hearing aids, somewhere between 1·5:1000 and 2:1000. The 1:1000 figure attaches to a severity of 50 dB HTL or greater, in the better-hearing ear. In the sample, children who had received neonatal intensive care were much more likely to have such an impairment (1:174) than other children (1:1278). Also, given some hearing impairment, they were much more likely to have further congenital abnormalities of a disabling kind. Over one tenth of the children identified by the age of three had an acquired impairment (including the progressive and the post-meningitic) but in the small profoundly impaired subset the proportion denoted 'acquired' was twice this. These epidemiological findings translate directly into service implications, such as the appropriate basing of at-risk screening on neonatal intensive care. Supplementing this gross risk indicator with presence of a family history increases the relative risk in the combined at-risk group to over 10:1.

The 1:1000 figure recurs very often in the literature and is certainly useful. Given the small size of the studies composing that literature, the probably heterogeneous populations and the poorly specified referral and inclusion criteria, the agreement between a number of studies producing a figure close to 1:1000 may even be suspiciously high. Several studies together suggest a total figure of about 3·5 or four per thousand known by school age to have at least a mild permanent hearing loss, including unilateral cases.[1] This raises again the issue of which children are appropriate targets of screening, and which should be referred when suspected of having a hearing problem. (Though related, these two criteria are not identical). Conditions, or degrees of severity, to be deliberately screened for must comprise clear cases of ability to benefit from a regime of treatment or (re)habilitation such as hearing aids. On the other hand, counselling and awareness of special educational needs can be reasonably offered not only to such cases but also to mild cases detected on a reactive (symptomatic) basis or incidentally detected by a screen.

Research could offer more precise criteria of candidature for intervention in congenital cochlear impairment. This has not yet been done for several reasons: (i) lack of any evident harm from incidental correct detections of the mildest cases, even if on the margin benefit to development and performance is in doubt; (ii) the relatively flat prevalence-severity distribution, entailing that only relatively small differences in numbers follow from ranging the lower boundary of candidature; and (iii) the usual statistical problem of the small numbers in any one centre. Point (i) amounts to a justification for a multicentre randomised controlled trial on hearing aid provision in children with **mild** bilateral cochlear hearing losses. The justification arises from the imminently changing circumstances; new screening techniques will detect a very high percentage of the congenital mild cases, as many of these will be covered by neonatal at-risk screening; they will also be found early in life, rather than across the first five years. As a pre-condition for recruiting cases, those professionals attuned to clinical trials as the means of escape from past uncertainties would need to agree upon the range within which honest and reasoned disagreement exists, or where the factors that bear on management and determine outcome need to be documented. As a general indication, this might be 20–40db mean HTL, on the better-hearing ear. By no means all such cases receive hearing aids currently. In the past, cases requiring help defined themselves by default; if mild cases did not present until late or at all the uncertainty about their treatment was not an issue. Now that many mildly impaired children can and will be detected early by neonatal screening, such a trial to guide practice is a necessary part of the proactive strategy. Given the flatness of the prevalence/severity distribution, this is not chiefly an issue of cost. It could be viewed as unethical to **fail** to conduct trials to determine the balance of risk and benefit in these children with mild bilateral cochlear impairments.

The consequences of a hearing loss are conveniently, though by no means comprehensively, predicted by a single variable—the hearing level in the better-hearing ear. Also important are whether and how the impairment deteriorates or remits over time, and the status of the poorer ear. Whilst many forms of hearing loss are broadly symmetrical, acquired cochlear hearing losses, particularly those due to infection or trauma, contain a relatively high proportion of unilateral cases. Evidence now exists[20] that these children do suffer some educational disadvantages although impact is obviously not so great as those of the bilateral severely impaired. Inevitably, as outlined in Chapter 2, such children will experience great difficulties when a soft sound to be attended to and discriminated is located on their poorer-hearing side, and also when noise or reverberation is also present. Unilaterally affected children emit inconsistent behaviours, appearing to hear well in favourable instances, but not otherwise, and in some instances orienting asymmetrically, but only the behaviourally sophisticated parent or teacher will infer the nature of the problem or devise the appropriate behavioural compensations. It is not clear to what extent the educational disadvantage in unilaterals may have been compounded by poor behavioural management of these children by parents or teachers, due for example to poor understanding of conflicting evidence. Generally, such children would not receive a hearing aid, although in the rare case of unilateral permanent conductive hearing loss, considerable benefit can be expected from an aid on the affected ear. Whilst unilaterally affected children could be found by screening, it is not clear that the degree of benefit they would receive from intervention justifies making them a main target. Hence including their numbers or the health gain for them in the justification for the screen may not be warranted. On balance, the existence of sequelae evidence suggests that it could be warranted, subject to demonstration of benefit from a specifiable intervention.

For severely affected children the risks and costs associated with detection are reasonably set aside as secondary. There is however an issue of undermined parental bonding with a child labelled at the beginning of its life as abnormal. This does not seem to be a major obstacle in families with neonates at risk who are already concerned or aware. Sufficient numbers of not-at-risk children have not yet been identified neonatally from universal or not-at-risk screening to be reassured in respect of them. For children with impairments that are unilateral or of marginal severity, the possible **dis**advantages of screening and confirmation of a hearing loss have to be considered quite seriously. These disadvantages could comprise: inappropriate (over)treatment, unnecessary anxieties for the parents of the inevitable false-positives, the encouragement of excessive dependency, identity problems, and lack of confidence or a failure complex through parental over-compensation or over-protection. Formal evidence on such personality dimensions is in short supply, but the rarity of evident harm done suggests that in the context of the present screening and surveillance system, the **dis**advantages from detection and awareness of impairment are probably not great. On balance it may be preferable to identify cases and counsel families against any such maladaptive patterns in the context of the increased awareness arising from screening. In general, decisions on screening policy involving the extension of screening into new problem areas have to be taken in the light of possibly diminishing returns for extension of the criteria of inclusion and the imperfectly known balance of benefits against disadvantages. However, in practice, the freedom to vary criteria for screening and referral is often limited by the properties of the technique available. In theory the criterion would be varied according to the subjective probability of the benefits exceeding the disadvantages for some tranche of individuals that would be differentially affected. For example, the oto-acoustic emissions technique has a markedly 'stepped' input/output function, i.e. it separates normal hearing (better than about 20–25 dB HTL) from all greater severities of impairment, but offers little gradation. In neonatal screening it therefore has a 'natural' cut-off that is rather low. This necessitates referral of all failing (or perhaps bilateral) cases for assessment to see whether the hearing level is really, for example, just over 25 dB HTL versus, say, 95 dB HTL (i.e. profoundly deaf). The very real ethical problem in the marginal case where referral (unfortunately labelled 'failure') may have disadvantages exceeding the benefits, justifies further research on such benefits in addition to the proposed trial. However, there is a difficulty with demonstrating absence of disadvantage. Very large, careful and generally costly studies are needed to demonstrate null results reliably.

In screening, the ears can be tested separately, or together. If tested separately, referral of unilateral cases could be suppressed (unless severe) at the screening stage, and anxiety and cost would thereby be reduced. However there is then the issue of a 'false sense of security' in relation to problems that may deteriorate or may compound later on. Increasingly there will be legal obstacles to **not** taking action upon information, however marginal, even where the benefits are questionable. Samples, biopsy tissue, test results, etc that could provide information, may need to be covered by agreed policies on when to erase or throw away the information unused, for example when other information indicates this to be justifiable according to established principles. The foregoing discussion illustrates that the cost of inventing, developing and spreading new health technology may be dwarfed by the costs of determining whether, when, where and how to use it. Without such research there will be casualties. Until this type of post-implementation research is done on benefits in real circumstances of application, given the decision to have a screening system at all, it will probably become medico-legally necessary to refer all unilateral cases and mild cases detected onwards for more full assessment and at least counselling. Awareness of such implications has to attend the main decision to implement universal neonatal screens, and the first few years of implementation have to include a disciplined and sensitive vigil for possible disadvantages. Decisions to implement are mainly decisions about the ratio of marginal benefits to marginal costs and the information has to be gathered accordingly. We have to distinguish here the economist's usage of 'marginal', meaning 'incremental', from the general usage, meaning 'small'. In audiology the term has a variant of the economic meaning and refers to a boundary zone, of uncertainty between what can pragmatically be viewed as normal and what viewed as impaired, and contains elements of both meanings. Thus it means a level of hearing between a level 'within normal limits' and the severity that is generally accepted as meriting concern and intervention. Services usually start out concerned with the most severe conditions. In the decision whether or not to proceed from at-risk screening to universal screening at birth, the wider scope will bring in large early numbers of marginal cases, partly because of the larger total numbers, partly because of the probable choice of EOAE technology.

The issue of marginal borderline need, benefits and risks may be over-shadowed by the issue of incremental costs: assuming 7 per cent of cohort to be at identifiably raised risk, an extension from targeted to universal screening would greatly raise the marginal cost per further case detected. In other words, among the 93 per cent of children not at risk, the cost per case detected would be very high. The raw numbers suggest a cost over ten times, i.e. $(100-7)/7$, higher than the at-risk cost as a starting estimate; the differing nature of the overheads, not yet adequately documented in field trials, could modify this factor somewhat. The inevitably large leap in marginal costs will require the further absolute benefits (i.e. the further health gain) from early detection of the not-at-risk cases to be carefully appraised and scaled. Against the low absolute cost of at-risk screening, the high marginal cost will initially look discouraging. However, the dilemma that this poses may remain concealed behind four other considerations. Firstly, if we assume the existence of at-risk neonatal screening, is extension to universal screening then a more cost-effective method of finding the remaining cases than some other arrangement occurring a little later in infancy, or is it at least of similar cost? Secondly, assuming effectiveness, does allocating the extra resources to give these further children extra months of aided auditory input **early** in life compare favourably with other ways of spending the total health budget? The possibly similar rights, needs and expectations for at-risk and not-at-risk children are not the point at issue, and the Wilson-Jungner principles must not be forgotten here. We have no single overall outcome indicator of human benefit on which to judge early intervention. We could include an element for savings in the education sector rather than in the health sector but it is not easy to quantify the education costs for a programme with no consensus specification as yet, and there are few precedents for option appraisals that explicitly transfer costs between departments of government in this way. However, there seems to be some time in hand for this health-economic work to be done. It would take five years for the paediatric hearing aid and rehabilitation services to prepare on a national scale for the intensive work with babies required by ubiquitous at-risk neonatal screening, and hence to be able to move to universal neonatal screening. Thirdly a delay will also be incurred during the execution of research to establish the **degree** of additional advantage from neonatal detection, as opposed to detection at one year, for those hearing-impaired children not readily establishable as at risk. This major aspect of health gain at stake in any decision to proceed to universal neonatal screening dwarfs the mere demonstration of feasibility and effectiveness, which is difficult enough. Fourthly, the skills required for early (re)habilitation are high for reasons of difficulty in technique, and they are in short supply. It may well be cost-effective to apply such higher skills in more concentrated form early in life rather than diluted across childhood, although this idea will be hard to establish with firm evidence. Again invoking the Wilson-Jungner principles, we have to put a reasonable (re)habilitation service in place based broadly on such an assumption, before it can become ethical to install and evaluate screening of the not-at-risk on a large scale. I am not convinced that we are yet ready.

5. OTITIS MEDIA WITH EFFUSION (OME)

Otitis media with effusion (OME, or 'glue ear') is a term (like 'sensorineural') that deliberately loses a possible distinction. The distinction in question can be difficult to make in practice, and for some purposes is not necessary. Acute otitis media (AOM, or 'red ear') is the acute infection of the middle-ear cleft which may cause a build up of fluid (effusion) there. AOM is accompanied by pain and fever and is a common evolution of upper respiratory tract infection in young children. Secretory otitis media (SOM) can be asymptomatic in young children unless astute behavioural observation is undertaken; here the microbiology is variable and the infection, if relevant, is low-grade, but the sero-mucinous effusion continues without clearance. The effusion strictly only justifies the term 'glue' when mucoid and resistant to natural clearance via the eustachian tube. Such highly viscous effusions are often found in the persistent cases coming to surgery and have so come to determine the vernacular name for the whole syndrome of SOM: 'glue ear' which implies in a misleading way that all cases are of concern for persistent and material hearing loss. Whatever the composition or viscosity of the fluid, its quantity is what chiefly determines the degree of hearing loss, at least up to the point where the middle ear is full to the top of the eardrum. Beyond that point the determinants of the greater hearing losses among the range of losses possible with OME are obscure. AOM often leads to SOM, and the particular children vulnerable to one are vulnerable to the other, most of the risk factors being common to both. Most OME is in fact SOM, but 'OME' is a useful term that has taken over largely from SOM. The condition requiring to be detected and treated is a **future history** of SOM, but this can only be predicted from the past history and even then only impefectly. In this history AOM is a component and valid predictor, and SOM itself is a fluctuating manifestation, so the term 'OME', which does not preclude AOM, is used here, except where reports of treatment on specific diagnostic groups are concerned.

The above account of the difficulties of terminology may already have risked confusing the reader, but OME causes even greater confusion among parents and professionals. This happens primarily because of the very high prevalence, the varying severity, and the fluctuating, eventually remitting, natural history. These properties make OME sit uneasily with the principles of screening. At first sight the problem does not lie in the availability of acceptable and effective treatments. After some years of controversy, it has now been shown that antibiotics, when the course is properly followed, are effective against AOM. The role of antibiotics in OME is controversial; any benefit certainly seems short-lived. Other medical treatments such as antihistamines and mucolytics have not been shown to be effective against SOM, although they are still widely prescribed. Surgery involving an incision in the ear drum (myringotomy), aspiration of the fluid and placement of a ventilation tube (grommet) is certainly effective, in the narrow sense of keeping the ear free of fluid. So long as the grommet is in place and unblocked (usually six–nine months), near-normal hearing is maintained. There is no evidence that the grommet assists the long-term course or remission of the disease, although adenoidectomy appears to do so.[21]

The extent of medium-term benefit to the general communicative status and development of the child or to the family's quality of life from grommet insertion remains uncertain. No sufficiently powerful trials have been undertaken with appropriate outcome measures, although some small trials have produced null results. The need to do such trials depends on whether the condition causes a material deficit in the first place. There is not space here for a balanced summary of all the specialised evidence on developmental sequelae, but inference from indirect evidence plus the best direct evidence[1] suggests that persistent OME in early childhood does slightly retard the development of language, attention and communication skills. It also suggests that the hearing loss in OME is indeed the main channel of causation; other causes could include non-specific congenital pre-disposition to infections, possibly correlated with some aspect of functioning of the central nervous system, or with non-specific illness effects upon behaviour and education. Some role for non-specific effects in OME sequelae can by no means be ruled out, but it does not in general undermine the importance of the auditory deprivation argument; other effects arising systemically e.g. days off school could compound the auditory deprivation effect in synergistic fashion. The maintenance of near-normal hearing in the early years should be beneficial in early-mid childhood to these various functions. The important questions are: (a) whether deficits in these functions result from OME alone, rather than its combination with other influences, and (b) whether a group of children can be defined as to persistence, severity and synergistic factors in whom material sequelae effects and reduction in these sequelae from treatment can be shown in the longer term. These questions are answerable only through analysis of data from a longitudinal study of a type never yet undertaken.

Difficulties arise with the intervention strategy for OME, because surgical treatment is costly, not totally free of trauma and risk, and has side-effects. It is now clear that maintenance of hearing through repeated ventilation tube insertion leads to minor long-term pathology of the eardrum.[22] The hypothesis of early sensory deprivation retarding development implies that the persistent cases should be the chief targets of detection and intervention in the **early** years of life. Yet it is precisely these children in whom repeat operations would be required. There is an even greater logical inconsistency in the relation of present practice to the rationale for intervention as a means to secondary prevention of delay in language development: the highest rate of operations in the UK currently falls at about four to seven years, whereas the highest prevalence of OME occurs from one to five years.

Given that OME is so complex in its natural history and so enigmatic as to sequelae and treatment, should it be side-lined and the attention of otologists and audiologists turned to clearer and more pressing problems? That course is not defensible for several reasons, of which the most important are:

(a) The condition is of very high prevalence, and in its extreme and persistent forms can cause great concern to parents at the level of concurrent attention and behaviour problems, even if the evidence on speech and language are sometimes overplayed by the professional providers of related services.

(b) The typical hearing loss when fluid in the ear, about 20 dB HTL, may appear mild by the standards of the common symmetrical, gradually sloping cochlear hearing losses in adults. However four considerations argue for revising the disability implications of this audiometric anchor point upwards: the effect on auditory learning will be greater than on the exercise of learned skills; the hearing losses are often asymmetrical, which may be a cause of specifically disordered development of binaural hearing;[23] the type of hearing loss usually found, with its slightly greater loss at low and high frequencies, is more destructive to speech reception than other forms with the same mean hearing threshold level; and conductive losses are more auditorily disabling than cochlear hearing losses where sounds up to conversational level are concerned.[8]

(c) The level of surgical intervention is very high in OME, cumulatively up to 10 per cent of children in some districts, so the total costs of assessment and treatment (plus, in some districts, related screening) are also high. OME is the most common single reason for an operation, and the most common cause of hospitalisation in childhood. No detailed health-economic study of OME has been published for the UK, as the relevant data come from multiple sources and are not recorded in easily accessible form. However, OME is probably costing the NHS £30m in surgical costs[24] and around £200m per year overall, once the involvements of health visitors, GPs, clinical medical officers, school screeners, paediatricians, audiologists and ENT surgeons have been totalled. Although changes in practice might not affect all of these components, their multiplicity and the total bill contribute to the case for better research on causes, prevention and treatment.

(d) Research on outcomes does not yet enable us to say whether the general intervention level in OME is too low or too high, but it is highly variable from place to place.[25] Although the relevant considerations in the pattern of clinical presentation are not disputed, explicit consensus has yet to be reached on the criteria for intervention—i.e. on just which children are candidates for the operations. Even if the average intervention level were shown to be about right, it is likely that many children who could benefit do not receive the operation and *vice versa*. The considerable literature on clinical trials provides little help on the crucial issue of candidature and has failed to address many of the other relevant questions.[24,26] For example, the relevant outcome from surgery for OME is not the hearing levels, which we know are improved over the short term, but is a mixture of the language communication, cognitive skills and the behavioural manifestations of OME that cause concern to parents.

The fact that there are tangible and common side-effects of surgery in OME, albeit of uncertain importance, makes it essential to develop intervention criteria that are justified by evidence. It also enhances the case for seeking supplementary or alternative types of treatment, including behavioural management for some cases at least. 'Mechanical' approaches underwent a long period of neglect due to unfavourable trial results for auto-inflation, a procedure where children blow up balloons through one nostril. Now such methods are being re-considered, one study having showed a small beneficial effect; significant results of material magnitude have yet to be reported. Basic treatment issues in OME still contain many uncertainties, and it is sobering that so much remains to be learned about a condition of such high prevalence. Although many sceptics can be found among otologists and other relevant professionals, the balance of opinion among them goes in favour of fairly aggressive intervention in OME. This is true also among voluntary pressure groups, although a reaction to precipitate un-counselled surgery has now set in among health-aware parents. I have acknowledged that there are shortcomings in the evidence on sequelae and on benefits from intervention. The reader will note that despite being quoted out of context (*Sunday Times* 30 November, 1992) as apparently opposing grommet operations, I am only a mild sceptic and see the problem as one in case-finding and assessment, to separate those children receiving negligible health gain from those receiving material gain from the operation. The large numbers affected make the separation worthwhile. However in the absence of objective evidence from trials on the relevant issues in intervention[24,26] it is worth applying what is already known, so as to reduce the variations in practice that appear to be a large source of inefficiency in the system for delivery of health care.

Fundamental understanding of the cellular and immunological basis of the excessive immune reaction that creates the sero-mucinous fluid can be expected to lead in the long term to improved medical treatments for OME, but the timing of such developments is highly uncertain. Meanwhile, improved **selective** case-finding and criteria for intervention offer the major possibilities for enhancing the health gain, by redistributing the considerable resources that will inevitably continue to be applied to this condition. The challenge of the research required to tidy up some of the confusion is great. The advent of contracting between purchasers and providers of services offers a framework for introducing at least broad criteria for candidature, on a more far reaching basis than unenforceable 'good practice' has done in the past.

There are a number of useful electro-acoustic techniques for detecting OME such as the measurement of middle-ear compliance (tympanometry). However there has been widespread and repeated acknowledgement that it is not economically viable in health terms to introduce mass screening for fluid in the ears.

This applies to the prevalence plateau from about two to six years. The reason for rejection of a mass-screening approach lies in the fluctuating nature of the condition—some children will be in temporary remission on the arbitrary day of screening, whilst the 10–20 per cent failing on that particular day will require a variable but in total large number of re-tests to establish the persistence of the condition. A single test result does not predict well which children would fail many times. Other information may in principle be able to predict that, and the near future may offer a prediction model working well enough in practice to rival the overall performance achievable by mass screening on several occasions. Again, this requires detailed and expensive longitudinal research. It is regrettable that technologically-driven articles still appear on the detection of fluid in the ear in general practice implicitly assuming that all such detections are desirable from a public health point of view. By failing to deny the false implication, such writings serve to spread it. Were a low-cost, low-risk highly-effective treatment to become available in future, this caution on resource grounds against mass screening for OME might be softened. But the inadequacy of evidence favouring antibiotic treatment for OME leaves the time still far off when mass screening for OME could be encouraged.

It is evident from the fluctuating history of OME that the conceptual prevalence-severity distribution for OME has to include, if not be replaced by, a prevalence-persistence distribution[27] as in Figure 3.2. Whether severity in the usual sense of average hearing level can be practicably taken into account in producing such population statistics is still unclear. Measures of hearing level in the individual case are useful in reflecting both the general form of the disease and its impairing effects, and hence in contributing to candidature for treatment. However, the hearing levels for a fluid-filled ear can vary from 0 to 50 dB HTL. Basing a screen on raised (poor) hearing levels rather than on disease presence would still not dispel the enigmas that make OME rest uneasily with the principles of screening. OME therefore does not directly contribute a supplementary justification for having a combined mass screen of hearing at $2\frac{1}{2}$ to $3\frac{1}{2}$ years that would also serve to detect any cochlear impairments not detected by that age. Such a combined screen could turn out to have merits, but a great confusion of rationale potentially arises in combining a screen for persistent

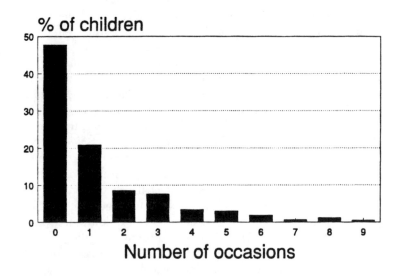

% of children

Number of occasions

FIGURE 3.2 The persistence/severity distribution for OME at age 2–4 years. The data was derived in a collaborative re-analysis by Stephenson *et al.* (Reference 27) from the Nijmegen cohort data. The definition of OME used is bilateral flat tympanograms (Type B) indicating that both ears have a substantial amount of fluid in. Over 1000 children were tested 3-monthly on 9 occasions. The usual clinical criteria for intervention emphasise **consecutive** separated occasions after an arbitrary entry point and must produce very high prevalences in a population study (18·2% here), of which any actual clinical referrals may be a somewhat arbitrary subset. In contrast, these population data emphasise the medium-term persistence of the history. It can be seen that in 69% of cases, OME was absent or fleeting. In 7·3% of cases it was present for at least half of the entire time. This is probably the most appropriate representation of the target group for interventions, which is still very large. In practice it is not yet possible to aim an intervention strategy at precisely this group, because those history or test variables that would predict membership of the group have not yet been established with sufficient accuracy. In other words, unless a 'screen' were to embrace up to 3 or 4 serial tympanometric test occasions, with at least 2 for those children clear on the first occasion, there can be no screening test for the target condition—persistence of OME. In practice the solution will come with a predictive test for persistent OME.

OME cases (nominal prevalence 50:1000) with one for **severe** cochlear hearing impairment (nominal prevalence about 0·5:1000). Equally we should be prepared for major tensions in the different technique requirements for target conditions so different in nature and separated by a hundredfold factor in prevalence. One possibility might be to define two separate at-risk groups at this age, one for cochlear hearing impairment and one for persistent OME. In this way a manageably small proportion of the population, those at materially raised risk for either condition, might be tested selectively. For both, the risk factors should include, but should not be limited to, suspicion-raising patterns of signs and history in general child health surveillance.

The variation of hearing levels in fluid-filled ears contributes to some asymmetry of hearing in children with OME. Considerable asymmetry is also displayed in whether or not any fluid is present,[27] particularly in population samples rather than in clinical samples. Having one ear hearing relatively well is advantageous for single faint sound sources in conditions free from noise and reverberation, but the advantage falls away when noise is present. Effects of OME on binaural hearing may have a long-term developmental implication, as well as a short-term implication for language input in sub-optimal acoustic conditions. Several pieces of evidence from physiological studies in animals suggest that the binaural localisation of sounds, and hence the adult capacity to profit from stereophony in separating wanted from unwanted sound sources in noisy conditions, is learned early in life; also that symmetrical hearing favours this learning. OME, and specifically the related asymmetries of hearing, affect the ability to use the important cue of spatial separation to distinguish signals from noise.[23] To some extent any deficit in this early learning may be reversed in subsequent learning, but it is uncertain whether this is due to a developmental effect (incompletely reversible effect of auditory deprivation in the early learning period) or to permanent minor pathology of the middle ear arising from the neuro-developmental disease and/or the side-effects of its treatment mentioned earlier. Controls for continued otopathology have to be stringent before neuro-developmental deprivation effects can be validly invoked.

From the point of view of arguments for early and repeated intervention to normalise hearing in OME, the implications from experimental research on binaural hearing are therefore three-edged: (i) It is probably important to maintain not merely some near-normal hearing, but symmetrical hearing in OME affecting the early years of life; (ii) Operating on a **single** ear will reduce total risk for eardrum pathology, but it may lead to temporary deficits in the ability to localise sounds and to spatially separate signals from noise (for example in a noisy classroom), and a bal-

TABLE 3.4 *An agenda for clinical research and HSR in children's hearing problems*

A. Pre-lingual Sensory Hearing Impairment

1. Further statistically controlled evaluation of the benefits of early detection and aiding in at-risk children with diverse and multiple outcome measures.

2. Trial implementation of neonatal screening on a universal basis having regard for coverage, costs and possible disadvantages. Supply of children subjects into (3).

3. Statistically controlled study of risks and benefits of early detection in **not-at-risk** children.

4. Randomised controlled trial of aiding/not aiding in mild-moderate hearing losses, using high-fidelity hearing aid technology.

5. Health-economic study of the benefits of cochlear implants provided early in life.

B. Otitis media with effusion

1. Multi-outcome randomised controlled trial of benefit of surgery in pre-school children to reducing language delay and other neurodevelopmental delay, behaviour disorder and illness symptoms.

2. Large longitudinal study of risk factors and natural history to provide predictive index for most persistent cases of OME.

3. Trial of behavioural intervention (training parents) in reducing cognitive and behavioural sequelae.

4. Controlled trial of new medical treatments in OME: steroids, antibiotics, hearing aids.

5. Estimate of under-referral of OME in families not culturally attuned to hearing problems.

ance may have to be struck; (iii) Inserting grommets in both ears is looked upon as a way of maximising the chance that at least one inserted tube (grommet) will stay in place in one ear (the currently prevailing view). However, symmetrical hearing may need to be positively confirmed after operation and where there is high risk of blockage, or after each grommet falls out, action should be taken to maintain symmetry. It will be some years before these conjectures from recent auditory physiology and psycho-acoustics will have progressed through the clinical trial stage to become public health issues where estimates of benefit, risks and cost can be attached to, for example, the maintenance of binaural hearing. However, they provide a good example of how research on basic biological processes can be discerned far ahead as having potential implications both for good clinical practice and for cost-effectiveness.

In this chapter I have discussed the two main areas of concern in hearing impairment in childhood—early detection of pre-lingual cochlear impairment, and timing and efficacy of treatment for OME. In each area there are large and important HSR questions to be addressed (Table 3.4) which require a public health perspective. However they cannot be cogently formulated from that perspective alone. A mixture of scientific, technological, public health and clinical understanding is required to pose and answer the right questions.

REFERENCES

1. HAGGARD, M. P., AND HUGHES, E. A., (1991). *Screening Children's Hearing.* HMSO, London.
2. CONRAD, R., (1979). *The deaf schoolchild.* Harper and Row, London.
3. MOORE, D. R., (1985). 'Postnatal development of the mammalian auditory system and the neural consequences of auditory deprivation'. *Acta Otolaryngologica* (Suppl 421): 19–30.
4. MARKIDES, A., (1986). 'Age at fitting of hearing aids and speech intelligibility'. *British Journal of Audiology*, **20**, 165–167.
5. RAMKALAWAN, T. W., AND DAVIS, A. C., (1992). 'The effects of hearing loss and age of intervention on some language metrics in young hearing-impaired children'. *British Journal of Audiology*, **26**, 97–108.
6. CHAMBERLAIN, J. M., (1984). 'Screening programmes'. *Journal of Epidemiology and Community Health*, **38**, 270–277.
7. HALL, D. M. B., (Ed.) (1989). *Health for all children.* Oxford University Press, Oxford.
8. GATEHOUSE, S., AND HAGGARD, M. P., (1986). 'The effects of air-bone gap and presentation level on world identification'. *Ear and Hearing*, **8**, 140–146.
9. DAVIS, A. C., AND WOOD, S., (1992). 'The epidemiology of childhood hearing impairment: factors relevant to the planning of services'. *British Journal of Audiology*, **26**, 77–90.
10. WILSON, J. M. G., AND JUNGNER, G., (1968). 'Principles and practice of screening for disease. Geneva: World Health Organisation.
11. HAGGARD, M. P., (1990). 'Hearing screening in children—state of the art(s)'. *Archives of Disease in Childhood*, **65**, 1193–1195.
12. McCORMICK, B., (1988). *Screening for hearing impairment in young children.* Croom Helm, London.
13. WATKIN, P. M., BALDWIN, M., AND LAOIDE, S., (1990). 'Parental Suspicion and identification of hearing impairment'. *Archives of Disease in Childhood*, **65**, 846–850.
14. JOHNSON, A., AND ASHURST, H., (1990). 'Screening for sensorineural deafness by health visitors'. *Archives of Disease in Childhood*, **65**, 841–845.
15. McCORMICK, B., CURNOCK, D. A., AND SPAVINS, F., 'Auditory screening of special care in neonates using the auditory response cradle'. *Archives of Disease in Childhood*, **59**, 1168–1172.

16. ROWE, S., 'An evaluation of ABR audiometry for the screening detection of hearing loss in ex-SCBU infants'. *British Journal of Audiology*, **25**, 259–274.

17. KEMP, D., (1978). 'Stimulated acoustic emissions from the human auditory system'. *Journal of the Acoustical Society of America*, **64**, 1386–1391.

18. COPE, Y., AND LUTMAN, M. E., (1988). 'Oto-acoustic emissions'. In MC-CORMICK, B., (Ed.) Paediatric Audiology 0–5 years. Taylor and Francis, London.

19. KENNEDY, C. R., KIMM, L., CAFARELLI DEES, D., EVANS, P. I., HUNTER, M., LENTON, S., AND THORNTON, A. R. D., 'Oto-acoustic emissions and auditory brainstem responses in the newborn'. *Archives of Disease in Childhood*, **66**, 1124–1129.

20. CULBERTON, J. C., AND GILBERT, L. E., (1990). 'Children with unilateral sensorineural hearing loss: cognitive academic and social development'. *Ear and Hearing*, **7**, 38–42.

21. MAW, R., AND HEROD, (1986). 'Otoscopic, impedance and audiometric findings in glue ear treated by adenoidectomy and tonsillectomy: a prospective randomised study'. *Lancet* 1986: **1**: 1399–1402.

22. SHAH, N., (1991). 'Otitis media and its sequelae'. *Journal of the Royal Society of Medicine*, **84**, 581–586.

23. MOORE, D. R., HUTCHINGS, M. E., AND MEYER, S. E., (1991). 'Binaural masking level differences in children with a history of otitis media'. *Audiology*, **30**, 90–101.

24. FREEMANTLE, N., *et al.* 'The Treatment of Persistent Glue Ear in Children'. *Effective Health Care Bulletin*, **4**. University of Leeds Public Health Dept. (1992).

25. BLACK, N. A., (1985). 'Geographical variations in the use of surgery for glue ear'. *Journal of the Royal Society of Medicine*, **78**, 641–648.

26. STEPHENSON, H., AND HAGGARD, M. P., (1992). 'Rationale and design of surgical trials for otitis media with effusion'. *Clinical Otolaryngology*, **17**, 67–78.

27. STEPHENSON, H., HAGGARD, M. P., ZIELHUIS, G., VAN DEN BROEK, P., AND SCHILDER, A., 'Prevalence of tympanogram asymmetries and fluctuations in OME—implications for compromised binaural hearing'. *Audiology* (in press).

4

THE ADULT WITH HEARING DIFFICULTIES

WITHIN EACH DISEASE GROUP OR OTHER CATEGORY OF MAJOR NEED for health services, a great diversity exists both of individual problems and requirements. This diversity is not merely idiosyncratic, but is structured along obvious dimensions: severity, age of onset, age at consultation, etc. Severe hearing impairment has its most dramatic effects when it strikes an aurally dependent person such as a Beethoven or a Smetana in a productive stage of life. However, in numerical terms, the increase in longevity in the 20th century has located among the elderly most of the burden of auditory disability, and hence most of the burden of care arises with them. In advanced countries, much of the expansion of the elderly population and hence of the hearing-impaired population has already happened, but people over 75, particularly women, will provide a large and increasing proportion of all **severely** hearing-impaired people for some years to come.[1]

The reasons for consultation about hearing disorders in adults are diverse. In the younger adult there may be fear of a progressive disorder, hereditary or acquired; concern about noise-induced hearing loss; or concern about organic ear symptoms. As the onset of hearing loss can be gradual and insidious, it may not even be the main reason for consultation, but part of one of several syndromes in which initially dizziness or tinnitus (buzzing/ringing in the ears) co-occur. Whilst some conditions that include hearing impairment among their symptoms do permit specific diagnosis and treatment, in most, a balance of probability between various possible factors is the best that can be given. In the elderly, consultation is sometimes pressed upon the individual by family members in the face of much denial, and here the omens for effective rehabilitation are poor. Although specific reasons for

References begin on p. 107.

consultation do not disappear, they are overtaken numerically by grudging admissions of degenerative change associated with the ageing process. This defensiveness against feelings of stigamatisation builds upon a more general systematic under-estimation in self-report by those over the age of 50 of their degree of impairment. Additionally, lip-reading (or more precisely audio-visual perception) which most people employ, irrespective of their claims, offsets mild-to-moderate hearing impairments with remarkable effectiveness. Consultation is therefore conservative and does not spontaneously take on the pattern that might be optimal for early intervention and secondary prevention. Despite the tendency of age-related problems to be viewed pessimistically, such stereotypes, underlying late consultation are unnecessarily pessimistic from a rehabilitative standpoint. In the population, the numbers of people with a particular degree of hearing impairment increase steeply after age 50 (Table 4.1) so age appears increasingly in the list of imputed 'causes'. At the descriptive level of analysis this is acceptable, in the negative sense of implying that further investigations to seek specific causes may not be health-economically justifiable. However in the positive sense of attributing a specific cause, age (i.e. the passage of time) is an ambiguous concept. It is difficult to rule out some role for the accumulated insults of living, and a hearing loss reasonably attributed to some genetically-based faster-ticking biological clock affecting the ear would tend to receive the label 'progressive'. For this reason many audiologists avoid the term 'presbycusis' as being pretentious, and where necessary use the descriptive term 'age-related hearing loss'.

From the point of view of prevention, the issue of hereditary or environmental causation is potentially important. The answer here is unclear and not yet of great practical use. Of the environmental causes, occupational noise exposure is largely preventable and this has become a matter of awareness, health promotion, good industrial practice and Health and Safety regulations. In recent years high-powered amplifiers and personal cassette players have placed leisure noise on the list of hazards for younger adults, but there exists insufficient data on the numbers of people, lengths of time and individual levels of wanton exposure, for accurately estimating the population hazard. Partial preventability is seen, via judicious dosage and careful monitoring, for certain

TABLE 4.1 *Hearing impairment in the British population*

Age Group	Better ear (dBHL)			Worse ear (dBHL)		
	≥ 25	≥ 45	≥ 65	≥ 25	≥ 45	≥ 65
17–30	1·8	0·2	< 0·1	5·6	1·3	< 0·1
31–40	2·8	1·1	0·7	10·4	2·5	1·1
41–50	8·2	1·7	0·3	20·0	5·9	2·0
51–60	18·9	4·0	0·9	33·9	10·7	4·4
61–70	36·8	7·4	2·3	51·2	19·0	7·5
71–80	60·2	17·6	4·0	71·6	33·1	12·5
Overall	16·1	3·9	1·1	26·1	9·3	3·5

The prevalence (%) of hearing impairment (dB hearing threshold averaged over 0·5, 1, 2, 4kHZ) in better and worse ears as a function of age group, from the MRC National Study of Hearing (Davis, Reference 1).

Although British standard terminology locates the boundaries differently, the three severities tabulated can be roughly thought of as 'mild or greater'; 'moderate or greater', and 'severe plus profound'. The ear asymmetries giving greater prevalence for the ear defined as 'worse' is due to the partly random occurrence of specific pathologies, mostly those of the conductive mechanism of the middle ear. In the better-hearing ear (the major determinant) of disability and where impairments are symmetrical they are more often cochlear (sensorineural) in origin. As a rule of thumb, the prevalence drops by a factor of 2 as 10 dB is added to the inclusion criterion. This is the 'prevalence-severity distribution' referred to in the text. A logarithmic function also describes age trends as well; for example ≥ 45 dB HL the prevalence roughly doubles per decade.

medically necessary drugs known to damage the ear (ototoxic). There seem to be only weak familial effects in general adult hearing impairment; this suggests some heritable differences in vulnerability to a variety of influences, and some polygenic determination of the rate of dying of the transducer cells in the cochlea. There is an elusive but probably real link between hearing impairment and cardiovascular disease, which is far from straightforward, and probably reflects an exacerbation of the effects of other pathologies by poor local blood supply. Viscosity of the blood is one of very few additional variables so far shown to contribute to the prediction of hearing levels of individuals in the population, once age, sex, occupational group and noise exposure have been taken into account.[2] The isolation of such predictive factors gives some hope for eventual prevention and for the development of specific medical treatments. Generally however, biomedical science has yet to strike at the roots of causation of hearing impairment, and treatment is largely denied the prestige of high-technology curative medicine. As a result, the main thrust of the service for hearing impairment in adult life is a check to rule out the presence of progressive treatable pathology, possible provision of such treatment followed by the provision of hearing aids and, in some instances, by accompanying rehabilitation. Before covering this more fully, I will discuss an important exception.

1. SCOPE FOR MIDDLE-EAR SURGERY

The location and scale of the organs affected by disease of the middle ear makes surgical treatment a real possibility, while the scope for surgery in the inner ear (cochlea)—is still extremely limited. Progress in surgical instrumentation and technique in the 1950s and 1960s led to surgical reconstruction of damaged middle ears on a wide scale in the 1960s and 1970s. Two chief diseases, otosclerosis and chronic suppurative otitis media are involved. Otosclerosis is an abnormality of bone growth, which immobilises the small chain of bones in the middle ear that couple the inner ear to the outside air pressure changes comprising sound. Chronic otitis media (COM) in adults is inflammation of the middle ear leading to degeneration of the eardrum and connecting bones, plus, in many cases, involvement of the mastoid air cells; this can run a very small risk of leading to a brain abscess. Although improved socio-economic conditions, including better general health and medical treatment have lowered the incidence of severe forms in recent decades, COM remains prevalent, partly due to increased longevity. Table 4.2 shows the gross breakdown, by category of hearing impairment, for the adult population of Great Britain, taken from the *National Study of Hearing*.[3] It also gives the prevalence of the two main conductive pathologies mentioned; they are by no means uncommon. The pathogenesis of both conditions remains surprisingly obscure; otosclerosis has a strong genetic component; COM may have a basis in a disorder of the immune system.

Both otosclerosis and COM can include some cochlear component to the measured hearing loss, although this depends on the spread of pathology. The predominantly middle-ear site of pathology makes the hearing loss chiefly conductive in form. Without a cochlear component the hearing level tends to reach a maximum at about 55–60 dB HTL, a moderate-to-severe impairment. This figure is a little more than the available gain from the

TABLE 4.2 *Middle ear disease in the adult population*
Entries are population prevalences (%) as given by Browning and Gatehouse (Reference 3). The four diagnoses are separated on the basis of the otoscopic, audiometric and tympanometric findings. COM = chronic otitis media. The diagnosis of otosclerosis is presumptive, on the basis of a normal eardrum appearance, but a gap between the hearing level by air-and by bone-conduction audiometry. The figures show presence of some significant middle ear pathology in around 6 per cent of the population, with a slight age trend; about two thirds have an associated hearing loss. Of those with COM, 86% had not received surgery to remedy the condition; 14% had received surgery but the condition was still active. There is thus considerable unmet surgical need in the population arising from middle ear pathology.

	Otosclerosis	Active COM	Healed otitis media	Eustachian tube dysfunction
Overall	2·1	1·5	1·7	0·9
Age group				
18–40	1·6	0·9	1·5	0·3
41–60	2·2	2·1	1·8	1·2
61–80	3·0	2·1	1·8	1·5
Sex				
Women	2·0	1·2	1·6	0·8
Men	2·2	1·9	1·9	1·1
Occupational Group				
Non-manual	1·5	0·8	1·3	0·8
Manual	2·7	2·2	2·1	1·1

transformer action of the middle ear, because middle ear obstructions can have the effect of clamping the transmission channel into the inner ear, not merely of removing its contribution. The middle-ear site is also accessible to surgical approach, with only small risk of serious permanent iatrogenic damage as a side-effect—at least in surgeons who maintain their skills on an appropriately large caseload. Since the early rapid progress in technique there has been a slight loss of interest in such surgery. This is only partly attributable to changing fashion. With any treatment there are usually high early hopes for high benefit at low cost, and optimistic assumptions about freedom from risk; these typically become moderated with experience, sometimes with an intervening period of disillusionment.

Middle-ear operations can have either one, or both, of two purposes: to arrest the progression of pathology and to improve hearing. The former is obviously characterised by secondary prevention; preventive aspects of hearing aid provision are discussed later. For operations that stand to improve hearing, a high standard is set by the risk-free benefit available from hearing aids. In middle-ear pathologies, benefit from hearing aids is high because amplification is an inverse of, and is hence a largely adequate solution for, the middle-ear attenuation involved. Also, for reasons of risk, there is some reluctance to operate on both ears, or on the better-hearing ear of an individual, unless the alternatives are very limited. The diminution of interest in reconstructive surgery of the middle ear has been accompanied by the supposition on the part of some ENT surgeons that the prevalence of otosclerosis may have decreased in recent decades. Given the strong genetic component, with most cases presenting after the age of reproduction, any such decrease is improbable, and the impression is more probably due simply to mistaking the backlog emerging in the 1960s and 1970s for a long-term high incidence, and to a slight loss of interest over the years as the balance of benefits to side-effects learn to be better appreciated.

Surgical improvement of hearing in both otosclerosis and COM may play an important part in a dual treatment strategy, by involving both surgery and a hearing aid. It can reduce the amplifier gain required in an aid (and hence both its capital and running costs); it also relaxes the tolerances required in the production of the anatomical earmould by which the amplified sound is coupled into the ear canal. This in turn reduces the very important practical problem of service delivery at the hearing aid stage. The tolerances widen for reasons of the reduced acoustical feedback experienced when using lower amplifier gains as may be possible after successful surgery, and this also increases the convenience for the user. (Feedback is the cause of the whistling that hearing aids sometimes emit when the sound output feeds back past the earmould into the microphone). The quality of earmoulds is an important service delivery problem in terms both of feedback and comfort. A high proportion of otosclerosis cases—higher than in the 1960s and 1970s—are nowadays simply referred for a hearing aid probably because of moderated professional optimism. Surveys have not been done to determine the typical appropriateness of the current pattern of referral. Detailed examination of issues of candidature and the balance of benefits, risks and costs from the various treatment options could lead to more sophisticated third-generation 'packages' of treatment, in which surgery and prosthetics are seen as complementary rather than as competing alternatives.

The treatment strategies in ear surgery and the delimitation of appropriate candidates have suffered from the use of a narrow impairment-based measure of treatment outcome—'closure of the air-bone gap'. This is the technical reduction of the conductive component of the hearing loss on the operated ear. What matters rather is whether functional hearing is materially improved. One consideration in outcome is the extent to which symmetry of hearing is restored, and another is the lack of iatrogenic damage to the high frequencies above 2 kHz, the highest on which the conductive component is conventionally assessed. The reader will not by now be surprised at my reason for taking a broader view of outcome measures and advocating them in the intervention strategy for, and in the audit of, ear surgery. The reason lies once again in the general importance of binaural hearing for separating wanted sounds from interfering noise. As the high frequencies are those most subject to head-shadow, they are an important source of cues to the direction of a sound source, and hence are also important in locating and separating sound sources. More generally, substantial deviations from symmetry, which tend to occur more at low-frequencies for mechanical reasons to do with the effects of disease and treatment, tend to compromise binaural hearing.

Two recent technical innovations are tending to reduce the hard-and-fast distinction between surgery and prosthetics. Since the early days of hearing aids there have existed devices that couple to the skull mechanically, rather than to the ear canal acoustically. These are specifically appropriate in particular patients with conductive hearing losses where active disease in the middle-ear prohibits use of a closed ear mould; this bone-conduction technology contributes significantly to decisions about the clinical management of patients with COM. However, standard bone-conduction aids have three disadvantages; an unsightly headband to press the vibrator to the mastoid for efficient coupling; discomfort and some long-term damage to the unfortunate scalp tissue compressed between the vibrator and the mastoid bone; and poor performance as regards acoustical transfer and frequency-response. These disadvantages are reduced in the recent development of the bone-anchored hearing aid, which vibrates a titanium plug screwed into the skull with respect to the aid's own inertia. Such new devices are always accompanied by some uncertainty about their crucial parameters of performance and the exact criteria for candidature. It has been shown that one of the two devices first appearing on the market had barely enough power to materially help the main clinical group that has the need for this type of aid; the range of suitable patients for it was determined in terms of the cochlear and the middle-ear components of the hearing loss and design changes recommended. The other device is, however, a more widely useful addition to the list of management options.[4]

In the wake of the bone-anchored hearing aid may come a miniature hearing aid coupled mechanically to the bones of the middle ear—the middle-ear implant. This is in some ways a logical step; in a standard hearing aid the motion of its miniature earphone is already mechanical, so transduction into sound for transmission through a few centimetres of air and then back again to mechanical movement seems perverse. However, there can sometimes be good safety reasons for using such indirect coupling, as is seen increasingly in the optical isolation of what would otherwise be hazardous links between people and electrical equipment.[1] As another example, television amplifiers for the hearing impaired do not plug into television sets where the high voltage for the cathode ray tube is close by, but use the less efficient airpath. Certainly middle-ear implants would need to have fail-safe precautions against over-amplification or malfunction.

An economic note of caution on the appropriate scale of application of implantable devices is in order here. I will not dwell on the psychological and cosmetic reasons for people wishing a bodily 'cure' rather than an obvious prosthetic badge of disability; whilst this cannot be allowed totally to override considerations of cost and effectiveness, it cannot be disregarded. It is highly likely that effective middle-ear implants will eventually be engineered and sold. It remains unclear whether, for large enough numbers of patients or patients with specific requirements, the additional benefits will outweigh the additional risks and costs. How could it be possible for a non-beneficial treatment to survive and spread? The US market for health care has been one of the chief stimuli to the development of medical technology. It is driven partly by considerations of cost and benefit; what can be paid for by whom, and how, are also important. Surgical operations are covered by standard health insurance schemes in the USA, whereas hearing aids are usually not. It can also be in the financial interests of service providers to offer treatment packages in excess of need, or with a cost somewhat disproportionate to benefit. Over-provision and over-pricing are not necessarily eliminated by market mechanisms, because full information does not circulate to patients and to insurance companies in the way that an efficient market requires.

In this discussion I have referred to surgical risk as a consideration in treatment strategy. This should not be mistaken for any belittling of the scope for ear surgery; all surgical and much medical treatment involves an element of risk, and the risks in ear surgery are not particularly high. The epidemiological findings show that amongst people with the two main forms of adult middle-ear disease, the proportion currently receiving surgery is quite small (Table 4.2). Taken with the earlier argument for integrating surgical and prosthetic management, these findings are encouraging towards either some expansion in the numbers of ear surgeons in the UK or the focussing of responsibilities of the existing establishment of ENT surgeons to spend more of their time doing the most beneficial forms of surgery. Whilst detailed criteria of candidature still need to be developed, based on the balance of costs, benefits and risks, the unmet need is considerable.

2. WHAT MAKES A GOOD HEARING AID?

The title of this section could justify a book on its own, because provision of a hearing aid can be 'good' in several different respects. Discussion of these respects illustrates the problems of delivering a good hearing aid service. The most obvious way in which an aid can be good lies in the electro-acoustic specification— low intrinsic amplifier noise, adequate amplifier gain, low non-linear distortion (except perhaps at the highest output levels, where this may be a cost-effective means of providing an extra level of protection against overload), absence of narrow peaks in the frequency-response of the acoustical delivery system, a wide frequency-range, the ability to use a directional microphone and to adjust tone-control according to short—or to long-term needs. Hi-fi enthusiasts know that to achieve any useful combination of these engineering goals involves both expense and difficult trade-off judgements at the design stage. In hearing aid provision trade-offs also enter at a second stage—that of choosing the type of aid for the individual. As some of the requirements may even be in partial conflict, it is necessary to judge how much each characteristic matters for the broad target group of patients for each design. The slope of the frequency-response (i.e. the amplifier gain as a function of frequency) over the mid-frequency range is usually thought of as a separate dimension of requirement from the overall amount of gain the amplifier permits. However, in the extremes there is a link: those with the severest losses usually only have residual low-frequency hearing, so may need anextended low-frequency response, while amplification at high frequencies can be pointless. Those with the more mild but aidable hearing losses require an extended high-frequency response but little gain at low frequencies. Once all the various mechanical or ergonomic possibilities for the controls are also considered, the number of possible combinations becomes very large. The unfavourable economics of small-volume production and stock holdings readily show that, in the planning of a service or marketing strategy as a whole, there is some reason to resist excessive proliferation of types. The great majority of needs—although not some of the rarer ones—can apparently be met with about eight basic types of hearing aid.

Each of the electro-acoustic properties listed above can be shown in controlled experimental conditions to yield some advantages to performance, although the differences are often small. Not enough is known about whether the magnitude of these advantages justifies the costs. However, among typical aid users, preferences between hearing aids are of low replicability and the obtained differences in performance are also small in relation to variability.[5] Furthermore, over time the brain becomes accustomed to imperfect hearing, and has to re-accommodate to the improved hearing given by a hearing aid. This is more than simply a matter of increasing loudness tolerance with increasing experience of the amplification from an aid, although that does contribute at the level of the user's motivation to continue. My colleague Stuart Gatehouse has shown[6] that the particular aid characteristic which gives the user the best speech discrimination only becomes determinate after a learning process of 8–12 weeks using a broadly appropriate hearing aid; the advantage from the ultimately 'best' aid is not apparent at the outset, so a limited set of comparisons is likely to mislead about which aid is ultimately best. To avoid confusion with other meanings that words such as 'adaptation' and 'adjustment' already carry, we have given this learning process the deliberately vague name of 'acclimatisation'. So far, the acclimatisation principle has only been established for the frequency-response, but it may be more general and apply also to distortion and dynamic range. The ultimately best aid for most individuals generally requires most gain at high frequencies (compensating the generally greater loss at high frequencies). Such an aid is usually not the aid that the user initially does best with, and certainly not the one most would initially prefer, as the unfamiliar sound quality is initially judged to be 'harsh', 'hissy' or 'tinny'.

The acclimatisation findings are of radical importance in three ways—one negative, two positive. Firstly, they show that direct **initial** consumer performance or preference is a scientifically inadequate basis for differential provision. In other words, if worthwhile extra health gain is to be sought by selecting and adjusting the hearing aid to the individual, beyond what is given by uniform provision, some new means of achieving this goal has to be found. (In North America, selective fitting is based largely on initial consumer performance and preference, after pre-selection of a broadly appropriate class of aid). Secondly, the results indicate that a more scientifically based service could result if the eventually optimum aid could be specifically **predicted** from characteristics of the individual, and if the selection and adjustment of hearing aids plus the related counselling were viewed as a 3-month evolving programme, rather than as a one-off step. This should be possible with only a small increase in the resources required for the initial predictive assessment and in the follow-up sessions required; such regimes will be under development over the next few years. Improvement in the effectiveness of hearing aid provision should result from taking account of the acclimatisation principle, but this will take some time to work through into services.

It would be a mistake to see the complexities entailed by acclimatisation solely as an extra cost burden to be overcome in the achievement of effectiveness. The findings on acclimatisation are also ultimately important as a scientific counter to cynicism

and apathy among professionals. The null findings on initial preference and performance as a basis for differential prescription
have hardly been encouraging to engineering investment in production of aids of high quality in a range of well-specified
characteristics, or to investing time in effective individual fitting.
There is informal evidence from the best of practice that such
effort is often repaid. In such circumstances a few positive findings
can be worth more than many null findings* and a potential
explanation for the null findings has now been provided.

There are other respects in which a hearing aid can be 'good'
or otherwise, besides as an electro-acoustic signal-processor. An
aid can only help if it is usable either extensively or in circumstances of importance to the individual. Its cosmetic properties
(particularly size) and ease of manual insertion and control of
functions in turn contribute to its use. The extent to which various
forms of rehabilitative advice and training encourage useful hearing tactics and realistic expectations has a marked effect on
willingness to continue using the aid in the early weeks. These
properties may contribute to subjective satisfaction with the
service received. However, much of satisfaction lies in the psychological characteristics of the user; it correlates only moderately
with measurable benefit. Part of this low correlation is due to the
imperfections of existing measures of benefit, which are based on
accuracy measures. In word—or sentence-based material, the
percentage of words correctly reported in the aided condition,
minus (or divided by) the same score from the unaided condition,
is usually taken as the measure of benefit. The use of time-based
measurements reflects the speed of arriving at a relevant decision
on the verbal material. Such a time measure helps to resolve some
of the vexing discrepancy between traditional performance
measures of benefits and subjective judgments of benefit[6] and

*Different interpretations of null results on preferences are possible, according to different
philosophies of medicine and health care provision. Subjective pleasing of the patient
contrasts with documentation of consensual benefits in definable groups of patients/users.
It will be evident from Chapter 2 that I consider patient-pleasing as necessary, but
insufficient. On an extreme subjectivist view, the patient needs **only** to be pleased; this
view leads directly to a bias in interpreting all but the most unequivocal evidence as
indicating that the nature of treatment does not matter. The task of finding performance
optima different from the preferred parameter values and demonstrating them must not
be underestimated; equally, the costs of demonstrating them and implementing them on
a routine basis need to be judged against the magnitude of the likely increase in average
benefit.

appears to reflect subjective effort, an important element in satis-faction. The time required to assimilate and use information is reduced in hearing aids that are reported as 'good'; there is also preliminary evidence that sophisticated methods of signal-process-ing that improve the apparent relative level of signal to background noise, without significant measured benefits to accu-racy so far, nevertheless show benefits in the time-based measure of effort. Despite this promising progress, it is unlikely that any single practicable performance measure of benefit can be entirely representative of the relevant acoustical and linguistic circum-stances in the lives of the diverse individuals requiring hearing aids, nor totally override the element contributed by their person-alities.

The suggestion of an ability to overcome the effects of auditory deprivation in adult life by early provision of hearing aids has been around for many years, jointly subscribed to by providers of hear-ing aids and auditory rehabilitation and by those of a more general preventive outlook. Any such effect is likely to arise not in the ear itself, but in patterns of neural connection in the auditory brainstem, and to be rather smaller in adults than in children. As remarked in Chapter 2, the major substantial argument for early intervention in adults may have to remain the duration for which benefit is received, rather than the eventual absolute performance. In the provision of hearing aids, the argument for early provision is perhaps even more strongly based on the greater re-learning ability and manual dexterity in a younger person, favouring ac-ceptance over the early weeks of use. Further evidence is required on the extent to which the ultimate level of performance obtain-able with a hearing aid may suffer, in proportion to the duration of unaided impairment; results in this area would provide the rationale for greater efforts focussed on early intervention to achieve secondary prevention. However, the delay and difficulty of the acclimatisation with an aid will also be greater the longer the duration of the impairment, and consideration of the respec-tive magnitudes of the effects may be a practically more important pointer towards early intervention as facilitating the overall suc-cess of a hearing aid service. The critical links to objective success are likely to be subjective feelings of benefit, realistic acceptance of limitations and incentive to persevere in the use of an aid in the early weeks.

Improved hearing aid services require progress on the technological front, particularly in aspects of hearing aids that reconcile
the limited dynamic range of impaired hearing with the
conflicting need for improved discrimination and selectivity in
noisy surroundings. However, research findings of the last two
decades also point overwhelmingly to the need to consider the
appropriate delivery of technology, to the extent of regarding
hearing aid provision as only the first part of a total rehabilitative
package.[7] Although some differences of emphasis do exist among
those who think and write about audiology services, this rehabilitation principle suffers more from inertial neglect than from
serious questioning. The deficiency occurs at the level of planning
of routine services, commitment to their development and the
supply of skills necessary to staff them. On these grounds I devote
the remainder of this chapter to the epidemiology of adult hearing
impairments and public health aspects of the hearing aid/
rehabilitation service.

3. WHO NEEDS WHAT?

The prevalence/severity distribution for adult hearing-impair-
ment in the UK is known to a high degree of precision (Table 4.1).
For present purposes, the type of impairment (cochlear versus
conductive) need not be considered; the cochlear type is much
more common, but is more difficult to aid successfully. It is usual
in an epidemiological context to take an average of the hearing
levels at various audiometric frequencies for purposes both of
statistical reliability and general predictive relevance. We have
used the four octave mid-frequencies 0·5–4·0 kHz; this avoids
susceptibility of measurements at very low frequencies to ambient
noise in testing rooms, and avoids an over-sensitivity to the very
mildest impairments, which typically affect mostly the highest
frequencies. The average hearing level on the better-hearing ear
is by no means the only determinant of auditory disability, consultation, take-up or benefit from a hearing aid; but it is the most
useful predictor of these quantities of concern that has been established to date. In the technical domain the average hearing level
influences in turn the requirement for amplifier gain and hence
for the need to control feedback from sound leakage round the
earmould. It also relates to the relative benefit achievable, and

to limits in absolute aided performance achievable. Beyond about 85 dB HL the numbers in the population are too small to estimate accurately by population sampling. For such small groups ascertainment methods have to be used, as for estimating the numbers[8] that are not helped by hearing aids but might be helped by a cochlear implant. Across the very wide range of about 30 to 85 dB HTL, hearing aids can be effective. The reality often falls short of high benefit however, and many auditory and non-auditory factors influence the actual benefit received.

Average severity of sensory impairment is linked to age, but hearing should be a more direct determinant of uptake of a hearing aid than age, on the grounds that the hearing levels are in some respects remediable, whilst age is not. Elderly people show an increased conservatism of responding criterion; hence their hearing impairments are not on average quite as extreme as they appear, but are accompanied by limitations in the central nervous system. However these contributory factors probably make the threshold as measured more rather than less useful because the limitations contribute to actual disability. The earlier mention of rate of response as an appropriate performance measure showed how speed and effort as well as accuracy of performance contribute to real world disability. However, the slowing of information processing by the central nervous system in elderly people and the related conservatism in responding, together set a limit to the maximum aided performance and hence a limit to the benefits a hearing aid can give. This limit is especially evident if expressed as a difference measure. These two related attributes however also increase the **absolute** need for some type of aid. This consideration urges that measures of benefit should also incorporate a **ratio** element whereby an absolutely small increase in information can reflect benefit to a severely impaired person who would hear little otherwise.

The public health issue as to whether, for a given level of hearing impairment, an elderly person would more appropriately have a hearing aid than a younger person, has to be faced in contemplating the scope for secondary prevention in adults or even the general timeliness of the investment. This has been left to individual factors in uptake, rather than to policies driven by health-economic considerations or to professional recommendation, for reasons which will become clear. The particular aiding requirements that are **specifically** linked to age seem to be few. Simplicity of insertion of a hearing aid and the ease of operation of its manual controls are the obvious example. Two size para- doxes should be noted at this point. The ergonomic requirement for large size, given arthritic fingers or other limitations to dexter- ity, stands in direct conflict with the cosmetic requirement of small size; noticeability, and hence large size, of a hearing aid may in the elderly also serve the additional purpose of eliciting helpful behaviours from others, such as slow clear speech while facing the listener. Although a separate consideration from the intensity of speech (which the hearing aid can in effect modify), the clarity and visibility of the speech produced are also relevant to comprehen- sion. An elderly person is less likely to need or be able effectively to executive sophisticated changes of an aid's characteristics according to the acoustic environment, but those might be pro- grammed to occur appropriately in an 'intelligent' aid.

In recommending how services should evolve, it is instructive to consider what group in the population currently possesses, or have at some point tried, a hearing aid, and also whether this pattern is optimal. In the early 1980s in the UK, the prevalence of such possession was 3·4 per cent. This is higher than anywhere else in the world outside Scandinavia, due chiefly to the service being free of charge. This is a national achievement justifying some pride. However, complacency is not called for, as the technological qual- ity of the equipment has not moved with the times, and the technical and rehabilitative quality of the service in many centres remains poor. From the point of view of health gain, even 3·4 per cent possession represents a two thirds shortfall in uptake (some of which may be due to underprovision). The justification for this challenging statement requires further consideration of who is an appropriate candidate for a hearing aid, in relation to who has one.

The concept of candidature is a vital link between public health and clinical provision, which is essential to medical effectiveness and to the functioning of the purchaser-provider relationship. In this belief, Stuart Gatehouse and I[9] developed a concept of candi- dature that was quantitatively justified by the large data set from the National Study of Hearing, complemented by clinical studies of the degree of benefit in patients with various characteristics. As variables to help define appropriateness we considered self-rated disability, patterns of consultation and evidence from performance measures on the magnitude of benefit as parameters: the 'best' distinction between candidates and non-candidates was defined as that which allowed two groups, not previously defined, to be most neatly distinguished in these parameters. The hearing levels on better and worse ears were considered, giving a two-dimensional space. For epidemiological purposes we have described hearing losses of 25 dB HTL or greater on the better ear (prevalence about 16 per cent in adults) as worth including in the data to be analysed. Among such people many may potentially benefit from a hearing aid. However, in our computations of candidature, the 'best' single criterion emerged as 35 dB HTL in the better ear (prevalence about 8 per cent in adults). This crite-rion was usefully supplemented by the inclusion of certain defined asymmetrical mild cases discussed below. The apparent conser-vatism of the revealed criterion is resolved by considering the chief purpose of having a criterion for candidature at all. This is to quantify need in the population, i.e. the gross **numbers** who **should on balance** have a hearing aid of the type at present available, in order to quantify the extent to which services are meeting a clear population need.

With 10·5 per cent of adults as candidates, and 3·4 per cent possession, only about a third of those we would describe as candidates have tried an aid. With an objectively derived criterion of candidature, the statement of a two-thirds shortfall in uptake or in provision of hearing aids becomes both fair and useful. One possible misapprehension should be immediately connected. Indi-viduals seeking an aid who have hearing impairments milder than this criterion should not be denied one, as it is **not** the purpose of the concept to say which **individual** may be **permitted** one, but to indicate a generally appropriate level of provision. Nor is the criterion intended to have an overriding force in clinical advice to individuals. For public health purposes, to lower the general criterion to 25 dB HTL would multiply the prevalence by roughly two, and make the small minority currently possessing an aid only about one sixth of all candidates as then defined. This would be too out of line with present reality, and not sufficiently supported by data on benefit to override that consideration. Such a lowering may become appropriate if high-fidelity technology becomes available to confer material benefit in such mild losses. The implicit allowance of a slight degree of circularity in applying

TABLE 4.3 *Audiometric and demographic breakdown of the sub-population who 'need' hearing aids*

	General Component BEA ≥ 35dB HTL	Asymmetric Component 15dB HTL ≤ BEA < 35dB HTL & WEA ≥ 45dB HTL	Recommended Criterion Total
Males			
All	8·8	2·7	11·5
18–60 yrs	3·5	2·1	5·6
61–70 yrs	19·8	7·3	27·1
71–80 yrs	41·5	1·6	43·1
Non-Manual	4·9	1·2	6·1
Manual	10·7	3·4	14·1
Females			
All	7·8	1·9	9·6
18–60 yrs	2·5	1·3	3·8
61–70 yrs	13·0	3·1	16·1
71–80 yrs	38·7	3·4	42·1
Non-Manual	4·4	1·1	5·5
Manual	10·3	2·4	12·7
Overall	8·3	2·2	10·5

The percentage of the adult population as given by Haggard and Gatehouse (Reference 9) in strata appropriate for seeking or obtaining assistance with ears or hearing. Percentages in strata are obtained by weighted projections from the National Study of Hearing. 'BEA' denotes the hearing level (0·5–4·0 kHz) on the better-hearing ear, 'WEA' that on the worse. The research established material benefit for the sample of patients meeting the dual criterion but not for others. It further showed that when a unilateral hearing loss becomes accompanied by a mild age-related hearing loss on the better ear (middle column) a hearing aid is beneficial and should be considered. The particular cut-offs were arrived at by locating a cut-off between those in whom benefit could be shown and those in whom it could not. The total of 10·5 per cent of adults who 'should' have a hearing aid (i.e. for whom benefits could be shown) defines a public health target for audiology services. When the fieldwork was done in the mid-1980s only one third of this need was met.

the concept has two important implications: improvements in the technology of hearing aids towards high fidelity characteristics, and conceivably some lowering of the related costs. This is also open to debate and further research; our work on audiometric criteria is not the end of the matter. Larger sets of data on the margins might provide a more refined formula, for example taking into account frequencies at which hearing loss occurs. But it is important to realise that our concept of candidature is essen-

tially a gross public health one applied to policy issues supported
by data in the mass. If need and health gain are to continue to be
driving forces in the provision of health services, and if resources
are to continue to be limited, a concept of criterion is inescapable.
We offer it not merely as an overall indication of the prevalence
of need but as a denominator for performance indicators of the
extent to which services meet population needs.

The fact that people have two ears is relevant to hearing aid
provision in two main ways. Table 4.3 shows that people with
asymmetric hearing losses contribute about one fifth of all candidates as defined. These are typically middle-aged people with one
fairly severely impaired ear of long standing, who then begin to
experience slight age-related hearing loss on their better ear and
hence are younger than the currently typical new seeker of a
hearing aid. Very few in this asymmetric group would benefit
from fitting the **better** ear with a hearing aid according to current
practice, as ears with 15–35 dB HTL are difficult to aid successfully—without taking a labour-intensive and technologically
expensive approach. In most of these asymmetric cases, the loss on
the poorer ear is largely conductive and hence a hearing aid on
that ear is able to restore a degree of symmetry of hearing. As
a consequence, not merely will hearing on the poorer-hearing
side be improved, but some degree of stereophony and binaural
summation will be reinstated; hence a high quality of aided performance can be achieved. Currently, this promising sub-range of
asymmetric candidates is not efficiently routed towards hearing
aid provision, and field projects on the value and best means of
achieving this are called for.

The second impact of two-eared hearing concerns the provision
of paired (binaural) hearing aids. Binaural provision has never
been dominant in the UK, for three main reasons: the greater
resources required, a technologically justified reluctance in some
patients to forego certain advantages that may remain in having
one ear unaided and, especially in the elderly a reasoned reluctance to have to cope with two small gadgets where one is difficult
enough. The idea that there could be an advantage in keeping one
ear **un**aided may seem to contradict the emphasis in Chapter 2
upon achieving functional symmetry of hearing for localisation
and attending to speech in noise. In the majority whose hearing
is broadly symmetrical, two hearing aids will lead, due to binaural

summation of loudness, to intense sounds more readily reaching the discomfort level, making the listener unreceptive for a while. Provided that group conversations, noise and reverberation are not often going to be encountered, a good two-part strategy can be to have one ear unaided so as to receive loud sounds with no extra distortion or circuit noise introduced, while permitting the other, aided, ear to handle fainter sounds; this avoids the problems and costs of the circuitry for automatic gain control. If group conversations, noise and reverberation cannot be largely precluded (and in active lives they cannot) then the advantages of binaural hearing override these considerations, and aids, matched to make the effective implants to the auditory system as similar as possible, become the solution of choice for those whose hearing levels on the two ears differ by less than about 10–15 dB HTL.

We have not estimated the specific numbers of people requiring two hearing aids, for three reasons. Firstly, in terms of candidature, the zones of applicability of the two opposed views of binaural aiding (boon versus encumbrance) are a little unclear. Secondly, there is an interplay with considerations of lifestyle, for which suitable statistical data do not exist and for which the use of age as a proxy would be unacceptably ageist. Also, most decisions on individuals will be influenced by the financial implications for the individuals themselves or for the service provider's budget. These problems of binaural candidature are by no means intractable; a considerable literature exists on their benefits, which is worth extending in the direction of lifestyles. A leaflet (Table 4.4) sponsored by one hearing aid manufacturer lists ten advantages for binaural aiding in vernacular language with the added vagueness of advertising copy. Manufacturers have obvious commercial incentives to promote binaural aiding, but the research literature on binaural hearing and aiding gives some-justification for all of these ten points. Perhaps regrettable is the lack of any mention of which particular people stand to benefit most.

By now it will be clear why the question 'who needs what?' cannot be addressed solely in overall public health terms; there are very good reasons why different people need different things. The health services research now required has to be driven by audiological understanding. This is not to say that the audiological research on hearing aids, particularly binaural aids, has successfully grasped all the issues; too much of it has failed to address issues of specific candidature and issues of cost/benefit or cost/utility at the margin.

TABLE 4.4 *Ten advantages of binaural hearing (and binaural hearing aids)*

1. *Safety*
   When a person hears with only one ear, the difficulty in locating sound can be dangerous, especially in traffic.

2. *Improved understanding*
   Binaural hearing helps you sort out and understand individual voices.

3. *Wider hearing range*
   A voice barely heard at 10 feet with one ear can be heard up to 40 feet away with two ears and two hearing aids.

4. *Restful listening*
   Listening with only one ear is physically tiring and stressful.

5. *Both ears stay active*
   When a bilaterally hearing impaired person wears a hearing aid in only one ear, the unused ear tends to lose its ability to hear and understand.

6. *Cushions loud sounds*
   Sudden loud sounds lose much of their jarring effect when divided between two ears.

7. *Better sound identification*
   Many noises which sound almost exactly alike when heard with one ear can be identified easily when heard with two ears.

8. *Smoother tone quality*
   Binaural hearing generally requires less volume, giving a natural sound to voices and music.

9. *Hearing from both sides*
   As nature intended, hearing with two ears allows you to enjoy a more normal social life.

10. *Hear with less power*
    Hear more quietly with less background interference.

There is a large and somewhat technical psycho-acoustic and audiological literature on the benefits of two ears. This commercial promotion by hearing aid manufacturers in the USA of binaural fitting (providing both ears with a hearing aid) summarises in everyday language the benefits that can be shown. Point 6 is questionable as expressed, but may arise from the lower gain setting that is required due to binaural summation. This is the basis also of points 3 and 10, and is mentioned as the reasons for 8. The leaflet in which the table appeared is relatively free of 'hard sell' but fails to point out that a minority of peoples' hearing losses are such as **not** to allow binaural aiding to confer any additional benefit.

4. WHY THE SHORTFALL?

The potential benefit from hearing aids is considerable, and the risk zero; even the possible damage to hearing from use of aids of very high power is contentious. The cost is comparable with that of common consumer products though in effect free to the patient in the UK health care system. Why then have only one third of appropriate candidates tried a hearing aid? As to individuals' reasons, no strong statement can be made but psychological opportunity cost may be involved. The epidemiological data on this point come from the National Study of Hearing, a general-purpose study that did not justify taking detailed measures of the psychological and social factors that are probably influential. We found that age, sex and occupational group influenced consultation, once the obvious influence of hearing level had been taken into account. Among candidates as defined in Table 4.4, male manual workers are least likely to have an aid. This contrasts with the fact that among male manual workers, hearing-impaired people (and hence candidates) are more numerous than among other demographic groups. Acquisition of hearing aids climbs steeply in the late 60s, around and just after retirement age. However on a broader age scale (50–80 years) the rate of provision fails to keep pace with the steeply increasing prevalence of hearing impairment as a function of age; so age-roles provide insufficient explanation.

Overall, there appear to be five interrelated main reasons for shortfall in provision or uptake, in approximate rank order of importance:

(i) Attitudes of both professionals and patients. Professionals may regard impairment as 'normal' rather than as pathological in the elderly, hence as not requiring intervention. Patients may erroneously regard the stigma or difficulties of a hearing-aid as less desirable than the cumulative adverse consequences as they attempt to pass off their auditory difficulties as normal-for-age, or as the fault of others, e.g. a general failure of the young to speak clearly nowadays. The contributions of these two attitudes can be distinguished, but they probably reinforce one another.

(ii) Supply. There is in effect rationing of access to hearing aids in the UK, despite there being no charge in the NHS. Although the service has training and manpower problems that need to be addressed, the restriction is due primarily and ultimately to resource control, and it works through many different channels— via the low number of outlets, and hence via waiting lists of a length significant in relation to the 'lifetime' of provision, via transport difficulties and the low availability of domiciliary visits to private homes or homes for the elderly, and sometimes via the reluctance of NHS budget-holders to provide more appropriate aids where those are more expensive.

(iii) Information. There is a lack of awareness of the benefits from hearing aids, of their appropriateness and ability to help most people with significant hearing problems, or of their availability free of charge.

(iv) Technological range and quality. Greater benefit is now available for some categories of user from aids of higher technical quality than those in the technologically obsolete NHS range. There is also a wider range of cosmetic options available from the private market, such as in-the-ear aids, which very few centres make available through the NHS; there are also aids for spe-cialised requirements. Alternatively this could be classified as an aspect of the resource and supply problem, (ii) above.

(v) General service quality and pattern of professionalisation. In most respects the NHS auditory rehabilitation service is **under**-professionalised, particularly in terms of the professional seniority of those responsible for developing it, those taking decisions on provision in individuals, and those providing rehabili-tation. There have been suggestions that many of the needs are relatively straightforward and that supply problems could be over-come by de-skilling and de-professionalising. These two views are not in opposition; if applied to different aspects of the system they can be reconciled. Many of the necessary patient contact hours in hearing aid provision can be appropriately provided by technician staff, if fully trained according to recommended training standards and especially if overseen by an audiological scientist or audiolog-ical physician with a specialised responsibility and interest.** In

**In the present system the pathway to provision via referral to an ENT consultant for a diagnostic check interposes inefficient delays. These are increasingly being avoided by setting up types of 'direct referral' system, with medical cross-referral available as a back-up; but these questions do not address the basic problems of the overall quality of the service.

an organisation large enough to justify some division of labour, **some** of the work would not need even full technician skills, and could be done by technical assistants. Much of the rehabilitative work can be done by hearing therapists with only rudimentary technical skills.

As a comment on the fifth reason for shortfall, extreme division of labour cannot be a universal solution, as it pre-supposes units of organisation large enough to fine-tune the mix of skills for components of the service. This justifiable complexity and scale is not consistent with the also attractive idea of solving supply problems by making hearing aids available on a more local level, which points either to smaller professional units or more mobile services. The division of labour also assumes the existence or creation of separate pools of trained personnel from which to recruit. In most parts of the country these conditions are not currently met. Neither centralised planning nor pseudo-market competition can guarantee to generate organisations with an ideal size of unit of aggregation for following a particular service model. It was recently put forward,[10] that the hearing aid service would be more effective if it employed lower grade and more briefly trained staff **as a mainstay**, rather than as a supplement. This seems to ignore the long-standing distinction between the limited technical competence for doing **much** of the work required and the professional responsibility for guaranteeing the quality of all of it. It also ignores the well-known psychological and ergonomic limitations to the fullest application of the principle of the division of labour.

Due to the inter-related nature of these reasons for shortfall in uptake and provision of hearing aids, a single or simple step cannot be expected to improve uptake or effectiveness of hearing aid services dramatically. There is no basis for imagining that some different economic system will miraculously transform the position. It is necessary to instigate work directly on all aspects of the problem, commencing with the aspects that are most likely to feed through to other aspects, or which are directly justified on other grounds, e.g. by the amount of benefit that would result from each provision. It is arguable that there **should** ideally be more similarities between spectacles and hearing aids, in terms of more widespread use at younger ages, greater cosmetic acceptability, de-medicalisation and provision via a commercial market.*** However, there are two important differences that limit the extent to which this is possible. Many visual problems are amenable to straightforward correction by an artificial transformation reversing that of the eye's lens defects; the appropriate inverse physical transformation is readily defined with high precision chiefly by reliable instruments which are only a matter of capital investment, and the optimum fitting is fairly clear to the customer. The same is not true in cochlear hearing impairments which predominate, where even the best frequency-dependent amplification with a hearing aid cannot reinstate auditory selectivity.

The genuine uncertainties in the choice of suitable aids have in the past been exploited in bad commercial practice to obtain money from elderly hearing-impaired people, while giving a poor service. This history indicates that an un-regulated private sector market might not be suitable for meeting population need on the basis of simple preference judgements and straightforward resulting consumer transactions, in the way that is adequate for spectacles in most instances. Some countries resolve this problem by separating the audiologist (whose professional fee can be standard, and who determines the need for an aid, plus its broadly appropriate type), from the dealer (whose income follows the quantity and value of sales and after-sales service). Making the audiologist more of a purchaser-adviser than a provider in this way is intellectually appealing, but it would not be the most efficient use of that scarce resource—audiological skills and would not help maximise health gain for the whole population. A role for the private sector could be ethically acceptable if the public health purchaser and the individual professional arbiter were financially separated in this way from the private provider. However, any such proposals would need to be well justified in terms of the

---

***In a wider context de-medicalisation in the manner of spectacles would increase availability in one sense: apart from the problem of high price this is roughly what occurs in the private sector. In another sense the higher price to the individual would then make hearing aids less available to the low-income groups where the prevalence is already slightly higher. Readier availability through direct referral or the private sector contains some medico-legal risk (of probably unimportant magnitude, if simple cross-referral criteria were followed) and some loss of ability to enforce standards. The latter is probably important, but for complex reasons high standards have not always been enforced in the NHS in the past either.

TABLE 4.5 *Agenda in health services research for adult hearing impairments*

---

1. Comparative evaluations of specified rehabilitation programmes for patients in various strata of need, e.g. severe hearing loss.

2. Evaluation of benefit from provision of hearing aids and evaluation of various patient contacting procedures for strata with potentially high benefit but low current uptake, e.g. mild hearing losses, younger users, asymmetrical losses.

3. Cost-utility comparison in conductive disorders of surgery, hearing aid and combinations of the two.

4. Cost-utility analysis of middle ear implants (anatomically coupled hearing aids).

5. Evaluation of hearing aid designs and follow-up adjustment schedules to overcome the 'acclimatisation' effect when attempting to fit the user with the best frequency response for him/her.

---

overall cost at which stated public health goals were achieved. The lower workload and hence the lower productivity currently seen in the private sector of hearing aid provision could mean higher real costs. Buying in the service from the private sector does already occur in the special circumstances of sparsely populated districts, but there is no obvious cost argument for extending this to general provision. Indeed it is precisely the bulk-buying power of the UK National Health Service and the full workload of hearing aid centres, due to excess of demand over supply for the clinical services, that helps to make UK provision of hearing aids so cost-efficient. Over recent decades, health and social security ministers of different political complexions have been lobbied concerning various degrees and forms of involvement of the private sector, such as voucher systems. They have all decided that the National Health Service should continue to provide hearing aids free at the point of delivery. This historical and audiological reasons for decisions and the related evidence may not be familiar to some managers and doctors, who may see the major form of provision for hearing impairment (hearing aids) as marginal in a hospital context. They would be content to let it depart. However so long as responsibilities for hearing aids and rehabilitation remain with purchasers, the economic analysis outlined above seems likely to retain service structures broadly similar to the present ones.

Technological, rehabilitative and public-health aspects of the hearing aid service all justify further research and developments.

However the mechanisms for implementing the improvement that knowledge from past R&D already offers and could offer further, also need to be strengthened to deliver a service better attuned to need, both epidemiologically and technologically. Issues of unit of aggregation, training levels, skill-mix and professional structures all deserve evaluation in health services research. Equally, technological forecasting has to foresee a wide and enduring technological plateau for the management of a particular condition (or a group of conditions) handled by the professional groups or the service structures under evaluation, or else the results may have too much built-in obsolescence. In adult audiology, effort will be better focussed for some time to come on the application, optimisation and evaluation of procedures, and on clarifying the distinctions between what is specific cost-effective treatment and what is minimal acceptable palliative care.

REFERENCES

1. DAVIS, A. C., (1991). 'Epidemiological profile of hearing impairments: the scale and nature of the problem with special reference to the elderly'. *Acta Otolaryngologica*, (Suppl 476), 23–31.
2. BROWNING, G. G., GATEHOUSE, S., AND LOWE, G. D. O., (1986). 'Blood viscosity as a factor in sensorineural hearing impairment'. *The Lancet*, 121–123.
3. BROWNING, G. G., AND GATEHOUSE, S., (1992). 'The prevalence of middle-ear disease in the adult British population'. *Clinical Otolaryngology*, **17**, 317–321.
4. HAKANSSON, B., LIDEN, G., TJELLSTROM, A., RINGDAHL, A., JACOBSSON, M., CARLASSON, P., AND ERLANDSSON, B. E., (1990). 'Ten years of experience of the Swedish bone-anchored hearing system'. *Annals of Otology, Rhinology and Laryngology*, **99**, 10(2) (Suppl 151), 86–98.
5. GATEHOUSE, S., (1992). 'The time-course and magnitude of perceptual acclimatisation to frequency responses: evidence from monaural fitting of hearing aids'. *Journal of the Acoustical Society of America*, **92**, 1258–1268.
6. BAER, T., MOORE, B. C. J., AND GATEHOUSE, S., (1993). 'Spectral contrast enhancement of speech in noise for listeners with sensorineural hearing impairment: effects on intelligibility, quality and response times'. *Journal of Rehabilitation Research and Development*. (In press).
7. STEPHENS, S. D. G., (1987). 'Auditory rehabilitation'. In HAGGARD, M. P., AND EVANS, E. F., (Eds). 'Hearing'. *British Medical Bulletin*, 43(4), 999–1026. Churchill Livingstone, Edinburgh.
8. THORNTON, A. R. D., (1986). 'Estimation of the number of patients who might be suitable for cochlear implants and similar procedures'. *British Journal of Audiology*, **20**, 221–229.

9. HAGGARD, M. P., AND GATEHOUSE, S., (1993). 'Candidature for hearing aids: justification for the concept and a two-part audiometric criterion'. *British Journal of Audiology*. (In press).

10. ROYAL NATIONAL INSTITUTE FOR DEAF PEOPLE (1989). *Hearing aids—the case for change*. RNID, London.

5

FUTURE DEVELOPMENTS IN SERVICES FOR HEARING-IMPAIRED PEOPLE

IN PREVIOUS CHAPTERS WE HAVE SEEN HOW NECESSARY IT IS TO study hearing and its disorders in the populations to be served, and to combine the findings with those from other types of study—biological or technological research. These two types of knowledge point towards the appropriate forms of service for hearing-impaired people in the health sphere. In general, a clear and stable picture already exists of most of the major service elements, if not of their detailed future form or best integration into a whole. This final chapter first outlines the course that two major new pieces of service-oriented research and development may take as we approach the 21st century. Next it returns to generalities, supplementing these two sections with a comment on changes involving the refinement of service 'packages' in which we would already recognise most of the ingredients. Roughly speaking, the first two sections are the province of biomedical and clinical research, while the third is the province of health services research (HSR). In the UK, 'HSR' has become the usual term for the type of care research in which pervasive issues of need, supply, demand, organisation, efficiency and effectiveness are addressed. Clinical research is most usefully defined as research on questions of detailed clinical strategy and tactics for particular health problems—what can be made to work, and how? The three activities—biomedical, clinical, and health services research— flourish most when closely integrated. Although usually progressing in that sequence, their development sequence from conceptual innovation through to mature forms of service may not involve clearly defined stages of transfer.

The requirement for formal evaluation that drives much HSR

References begin on p. 141.

can sometimes still surprise both politicians and some professionals accustomed to past modes of professional consensus, lobbying,
and constant service improvement from historically low baselines;
if the benefits require so much effort in their demonstration, does
this not question the entire enterprise? Should effects that are
marginal or debatable be left aside, and resources in research and
service be concentrated on achieving and exploiting radical innovations that are so evidently effective as to raise no such doubts?
Unfortunately two factors prevent matters from being so simple.
(i) New treatment regimes that would qualify immediately are few,
because initially the benefits can be variable and complex to
observe. First impressions may over-estimate or under-estimate
eventual benefits, so the latter need to be quantified in extent to
balance against risks and costs and against other demands for
health care. The successes of the past in the war against infectious
disease have helped to create a new profile of disease, wherein
further advances will tend to involve modest benefits, some costly
to achieve or to apply, that will hence require large well-controlled
studies to demonstrate them. (ii) Even where advances appear to
be radical, the ways in which they can be applied may be limited
by social or ethical factors; the new genetics provides a notable
example.

The need for designing and fine-tuning the delivery system for
health care is increasingly acknowledged. In the past it was
assumed that only professional knowledge was required, and that
this was automatically going to be applied properly wherever a
trained doctor and/or nurse were located. Nowadays the health
care industry absorbs between 5 and 13 per cent of GNP in the
advanced economies. Like any other industry, it has its contributing secondary trades, ranging from investment analysts to
educators, who assist the planning, delivery and fine-tuning of
routine activity. Research has an important role in this fine-
tuning, to which I return in the final section of this chapter.

Despite the above cautions, radical progress from biomedical
research and new technology permitting substitution or accelera-
tion of procedures and cost-reduction can make major inroads on
diagnosis and treatment of entire classes of health problem and
these are the major instigators of change and professional excitement. The present decade sees two major areas of radical progress
and expansion that are enabling services for hearing disorders to

escape Cinderella status, one an extension of medical genetics in audiology, the other in rehabilitation and the associated surgery.

1. MOLECULAR GENETICS OF HEREDITARY DEAFNESS

There is a familial component in the susceptibility to many diseases. Those which lead to the commoner forms of hearing impairment are only weakly familial. Given the multiplicity both of forms and of causes, this knowledge can hardly be exploited in prevention, diagnosis or treatment, especially given the statistical tendency to inherit not only the genes but particular environments. Some rare forms of progressive late-onset deafness are strongly genetic.[1] Several of the genetic syndromes involve a profound hearing impairment, and bio-medical scientists are not steeped in the conceptual and terminological issues in disability research touched on in Chapter 1. Accordingly, the term 'deafness' is more widely used in the genetic context.

Progress in the Biology of Hereditary Deafness

Of pre-lingual cases of profound deafness, about one half are thought to be genetic in origin.[1] Of these, a third (i.e. about 16 per cent of all cases) are either dominant or X-linked, leaving two-thirds autosomal recessive. This is the mode of inheritance underlying, for example, the high prevalence of deaf children born to marriages between normally-hearing relatives such as first cousins. In individual cases there may not be enough known instances in the family (particularly with contemporary small families and geographical mobility) to establish recessive inheritance. The estimate that one half of pre-lingual deafnesses are genetic is therefore made by statistical inference from studies done in circumstances most favourable to establishing the inheritance pattern. More typically, many individual cases of recessive genetic causation will be described as 'unknown', as will typically undocumented environmental causes such as cytomegalovirus in pregnancy, because it is not currently practicable to gather firm evidence. The disincentives to achieving true diagnosis in pre-lingual sensorineural hearing impairment have been effort and cost, lack of certainty, and a lack of consequent beneficial and differential courses of action.

The balance of worthwhile effort may be about to change, due to the spectacular rate of progress in molecular genetics. Any full appreciation of the new knowledge in molecular genetics of deafness would require some background in molecular and developmental biology, and in the pathophysiology of hearing. Given that requirement, and given the many different ways in which an ear can develop abnormally as a result of genetic abnormality, the account given here has to be highly summarised. A full review of the implications of molecular biology for the study of hereditary deafness is given by Steel.[2] In brief, the technology of gene mapping and sequencing is progressing at a rapid rate. Whilst only a small proportion of the genes leading to deafness have yet been located, it is possible with reasonable confidence to predict continuing progress in the location on the human chromosomes of those genes in which abnormalities cause or predispose the major inherited diseases. Once genes are located by flanking markers, useful genetic counselling becomes possible; the gene may also be identified and its DNA sequence determined. This knowledge allows the cloning of probes which enable the identification from human tissues acquired with minimum invasiveness (usually blood or saliva) of an individual's status as the carrier/non-carrier of a particular gene abnormality. In turn, a battery of such probes would enable the prospective parent with one deaf child or known deaf family members to receive much more firm genetic counselling about the probability of having a(nother) deaf child. The gain here lies in shifting the estimate of risk from those that are indeterminate or in the marginal zone where decision is difficult (e.g. 1 in 50) upwards to unacceptably high risks (e.g. 1 in 5) or downwards to a risk level little different from the background level (e.g. 1 in 500). Backed up by facilities for prenatal diagnosis, such technology offers short-term reproductive choices to parents. Increased biological knowledge is beginning to follow from identifying genes causing deafness in the form of an understanding of how the genes are expressed in development; this promises a better quality of medical care to affected individuals, and hence better quality of life (as is beginning to happen for cystic fibrosis). This is also a major reason for undertaking the genetic research. Some long-term possibilities of therapy by genetic engineering—repair by insertion of an un-damaged copy of the affected gene into the genetic material—even exist for some genetic disorders, although it is currently doubtful whether these will ever be applied in deafness. This powerful new medical technology merits some caution about the ways in which it might be used.

Social Implications

There is widespread awareness of the psychological and ethical problems introduced by the new genetic technologies, in particular of the dangers of a gradual slide towards eugenic thinking. Clinical geneticists are keen to do the relevant research on appropriate delivery mechanisms for the new knowledge, including counselling, and to set standards and guidelines. However, it may not be practicable to introduce regulations that would totally preclude mis-application, for example to ban commercial testing of individual samples in the absence of approved counselling support to families. Given some ethical caution and debate, moving forward can be encouraged, so as to realise the potential benefits from knowledge in an area where knowledge has been lacking. The ethical dilemmas cannot be gone into here in all their aspects, but a contrast can be drawn between cystic fibrosis and hereditary congenital hearing impairment that may be instructive. Cystic fibrosis (CF) currently leads to early death, a low quality of life, and a large burden of care. Support groups for families exist, but these cannot be described in terms of a culture or community of specifically CF sufferers themselves. For hereditary deafness, in contrast, few of the causal diseases affect the lifespan of survivors directly, whilst most have a variable but fair-to-good quality of life; the burden of care is medium to heavy and falls mostly outside the health budget. These diseases also repopulate the deaf community and hence recruit new members to the institutions that make such a major contribution to the quality of life for profoundly deaf individuals.

The way in which genetic technology can become appropriately applied in deafness will inevitably differ from the way that is currently developing in cystic fibrosis. There is some concern that the new genetics could be used 'against the deaf community'. It is necessary to examine what could be meant by this phrase, and to anticipate the likely evolution of events and conflicts. Deaf peoples' concerns appear to be threefold. (i) Value judgements made by hearing people, possibly based on limited knowledge of the deaf community, could be insensitively imposed upon deaf people, for example via value judgements about what particular reproductive choices are appropriate. (ii) Increasing applicability and application of a medical model, particularly in prevention, might make deafness become a more stigmatised condition in the future; for example, not to have avoided having a deaf child might come to be thought of as ignorance or irresponsibility by parents. The development of such attitudes would undermine recent progress in the elaboration of a positive identity for deaf people. (iii) The exercise of that reproductive choice would contribute to reducing the size of deaf communities further, to non-viability in some cases, unless better integration with hearing sub-communities occurs. Deaf communities are already heavily concentrated in large urban areas for obvious reasons. I pass no ethical, political or cultural comment either way from these facts and propositions, I simply report them in the belief that ignorance of them is likely to be more harmful than awareness of them. There are probably some sensitive contexts however in which it is unprofitable to raise these issues.

Professionals sometimes have difficulty believing those who speak for deaf people and organisations, when the latter say that deafness is not a tragedy to be avoided.[3] In relative terms, such a case could clearly be argued for deafness in relation to cystic fibrosis. However, in absolute terms a mutual misunderstanding then arises, because health professionals do not typically use the term 'deafness' as a natural category to describe a distinctive sub-culture. Deaf/non-deaf is a major dichotomous social category in the experienced world of deaf people, rather like male/female. In their view, insofar as deafness is a 'problem', it is a problem of and for society as a whole, to be viewed in terms of discrimination, opportunity, etc. To deaf people, deafness is not to be seen as a reducible or avoidable manifestation of various disease states, which are largely irrelevant. Professionals are not simply under-informed on the views of deaf people; rather, they base their understanding of the matter on the attitudes of the group closest to the problem with whom they can communicate— parents of deaf children, ninety per cent of whom are not themselves deaf. Professionals are also aware of the changing nature of the population of hearing-impaired children, described in Chapter 3. Early-detected children with well-fitted hearing aids can now make progress in units for the partially hearing in normal schools; few children are so deaf as to rule out this course in favour of signing and an immersion in deaf culture from the start. However, virtually all the professionals involved acknowledge that the adjustments of hearing-impaired children are diverse and difficult to predict, even with knowledge of relevant factors beyond the degree of hearing loss. So this understanding should not therefore be misconstrued as opposition to adjustment based on signing. These observations do not lead professionals to argue that the maintenance of a deaf population adequate to sustain deaf culture should be a goal of health services. Thus, whilst acknowledging the reality and validity of deaf culture, plus its value as a means of improving the quality of life for those who are deaf, professionals tend to favour solving or reducing the identifiable health problems of individual patients or their children. This difference of perspectives between professionals and deaf people leaves some room for misunderstandings.

A compromise position has been well articulated by professionals with specialised experience of offering genetic counselling to members of the deaf community itself. A service model has been developed for doing this in an appropriate way.[4] Chiefly this service must avoid value judgements and modify its presentation of information, including increased use of non-verbal methods such as diagrams and, of course, sign language. Such a service is the logical product of applying the following general principle to a particular risk group: that health services can only be effective if they take systematic account of the public's current views of health problems and abilities to assimilate information. Services cannot proceed on the assumption of major changes in health-related behaviours occurring in the short-term, even if such changes in the long-term must remain a goal.

Planning for New Services

The anticipated availability of gene probes for several types of recessive deafness is likely to transform genetic counselling by the year 2000. Despite such general confidence being justified by precedent in other fields, exact forecasts cannot be made of numerical implications nor of the timing of application of particular genetic tests. With the degree of diagnostic uncertainty reduced by a new battery of genetic tests, accurate diagnosis of environmental causes in children would become a more feasible and worthwhile enterprise overall, probably creating further benefits. Initially, the result would be a clearer picture of the precise causes of deafness, which would be useful for public health purposes. This could in turn contribute to better prevention and also to treatment in the medium term, through feedback on the occurrences and outcomes of preventable conditions and through greater accuracy of genetic counselling, using improved non-genetic as well as genetic information. The widespread misuse of the term 'diagnosis' for the confirmation of hearing impairment in a suspected child serves to conceal the regrettable lack of meaningful diagnosis at present.

We can anticipate what the requirements may be for delivering the eventual genetic counselling services. It seems unlikely at this stage that ENT surgeons or audiological physicians would broaden their work to undertake the genetic examination and investigations themselves as a supplement to their otological and audiological techniques. This seems unlikely on two main grounds: (i) some of the syndromes that include deafness involve diagnostic signs of and consequences of disease that require forms of diagnosis, treatment, counselling, or care that are quite distinct from matters of the ear and hearing; (ii) counselling on reproductive choice is a specialised and delicate matter. It seems more likely that regional or sub-regional medical genetics services will be supplemented by some sessions from an ENT surgeon or audiological physician prepared to specialise somewhat, but without over-escalating the training requirements. Non-medical counsellors will also be required for follow up, and it is unlikely that audiological, scientific and technical staff or ENT nurses would be an appropriate recruitment base for these. Parental feelings of bafflement, embarrassment, denial, guilt and several much stronger emotions, accompany the occurrence or diagnosis of hereditary deafness. The announcement of carrier status can contain elements of these coupled to difficulties of understanding the implications. Both require counselling by an experienced professional; specific experience is essential for informing decisions on reproductive choice and coping with the complex feelings that arise with the problematic decisions faced.

For most diseases the costs of diagnostic tests contribute significantly to the total costs of services. It is too soon to estimate precisely what the costs and arrangements will be for checking families with a battery of gene probes. The particular battery to be used in an individual case would appropriately be constrained by the general clinical picture and family history. This contingent approach appears not only appropriate but likely, unless the shot-gun approach of performing every conceivably relevant test for reasons of legal defensiveness, or charging by item of service rather than for informativeness of the test, comes to be practised in the UK. The tests will probably require special regional centres, Because of the costs of enzymes and other materials, a set of genetic tests will for the foreseeable future cost hundreds of pounds per case, rather than the typical few tens of pounds for current microbiological and biomedical testing. This arises partly because of the need to include testing of family members. However, the total cost of detecting, confirming, diagnosing, counselling and habilitating each deaf child already runs into many tens of thousands of pounds, leaving aside the longer term costs of special education. Given peace of mind for parents and access to better information than currently available about the likelihood of having a deaf child, the envisaged services are likely to be seen by the purchasers and providers of health services as cost-effective and cost-beneficial. It can be envisaged that the techniques will spread rapidly for two reasons, which are instructive about the forces which favour rapid change in patterns of health care. Firstly, medical genetics already exists as a professional discipline; though it can be expected to become more powerful and require further trained medical staff in the decade ahead, no major initiative is required to create some wholly new form of service. In particular, genetic testing will provide new ways of doing better what is already regarded as valuable—diagnosis. Diagnosis does not automatically entail high health gain, but clinical medicine is as much concerned with tangible implications as with ultimate benefit. Secondly, although the costs of the diagnostic tests based on molecular biology may turn out to be five to ten times the costs of conventional biological tests, the numbers of families will be small: the modest increase to the total care bill for each family should not constitute a major obstacle.

As long as the details remain sketchy the foregoing optimistic scenario for genetic services to hearing-impaired people may seem like an attempt to attenuate the demand for evaluation and costing that should be imposed on all trial services as they develop. Rather, these remarks summarise reasonable expectations based on scientific potential which have been used to give high priority to research that will lead to new services. The health services research required to implement the appropriate genetic services in this instance probably lies more in the area of health-related behaviour and health beliefs, than in the evaluation of effectiveness, compared to what we have recently come to expect. In this particular field, the attitudes, anxieties, understanding and uptake by parents, and the follow-through by the service will be issues of great importance. Part of this research can be straightforward, involving the counting of cases where various courses of action are taken, and the consequences for other parts of the health care system can be readily deduced. Other parts will involve the elicitation of more complex preferences and evaluative judgements. For example, until services become widespread, parents not receiving a molecular genetics service can be asked whether they might rather have had it; their responses will need to be balanced against the responses of parents actually receiving the service concerning whether they would rather not have known. As the judgements are hypothetical and cannot be made by the same parents (every individual is turned into a different individual by parenthood) the interpretation of this balance is not readily comparable in terms of quality of life with the interpretation of outcome indicators for other types of service.

2. COCHLEAR IMPLANTS

A little knowledge of the technology of cochlear implants is necessary to appreciate the issues in service development and research that it brings. The cochlear implant is a biocompatible electrical hearing aid that stimulates auditory nerve endings in the inner ear directly. It can bring usable auditory sensations to a high percentage of the profoundly deaf, for the majority of whom high-powered acoustical hearing aids provide little or no benefit.

Implants currently provide remarkably good results in a large majority of those implanted, but they do not 'restore normal hearing'. Normal hearing cannot be restored because restoring the complete time place pattern of nerve fibre stimulation is impossible, the full frequency range is not covered, and a very limited dynamic range exists between inaudibility and pain or discomfort through over-stimulation.

The State of the Art

The multi-channel cochlear implant was the success story of ENT and audiology in the 1980s and was depicted, labelled as 'bionic ear', on an Australian postage stamp. That term is misleading in a number of ways. High-precision manufacturing techniques are necessary to give the electrode array the necessary electrical, mechanical, and bio-compatible properties and to give its driver circuitry high reliability. Hence the hardware cost is high, around £13,000 per implant at the time of writing. The various external speech-processing circuits tried so far have all been fairly simple—and so far the more complex ones have not necessarily performed the best.[5] These **external** parts are closest to 'bionic' in emulating some aspects of the function of a normal ear, such as the compression of the dynamic range. As with conventional hearing aids, technological advances have initially been directed into miniaturisation and into robust specific solutions of standard communication electronic engineering problems—for example, general reliability and multiplexing the signals for the various electrode contacts with control signals to change the electrode configuration. In one type of implant these multiplexed signals are fed by direct electrical connection through a titanium plug set into the skin and anchored in bone. In another they modulate a high-frequency electromagnetic carrier signal that can be transmitted across the skin. In the latter the transmitter must have power high enough to induce a current that can stimulate the auditory nerve via the electrode contacts, but at the same time low enough to need only small batteries and hence to permit the external device to be wearable like a hearing aid. By comparison with electromagnetic transmission across the skin, the titanium plugs through the skin reduces the engineering problems, at the expense of increasing—but not unacceptably—the possibility of organic problems such as infection or damage by a glancing blow. In both types, a short biocompatible cable connects the receiver package embedded in the skull surface to the electrode in the inner ear.

Results with the first generation of single-channel implantees in the 1970s were unimpressive.[6] Since that first experimental phase four chief aspects of the technology and service have improved. (i) Patient selection criteria have been revised (for example by the exclusion nowadays of unpromising candidates such as people who have been profoundly deaf for more than a few years and, in particular, teenagers who have become a part of the deaf signing culture). (ii) Intra- rather than extra-cochlear location of electrodes has led to the stimulation of larger numbers of nerve endings and multi-channel design has led to a degree of discrimination in some patients between low- and high-frequency parts of the spectrum in many implantees. The spectrum is the frequency-intensity-time pattern that carries the phonetic content of the sounds which make up utterances. (iii) Increasing emphasis on, and professional skill in, rehabilitation (including counselling on expectations and support) has helped communication skill training to raise the overall efficacy of use of the implant. (iv) Improved surgical technique has avoided surgical complications. The current state of the art can be summarised as follows: material benefits from implantation of most patients are well beyond question, given the careful exclusion of certain definable categories of patient. In relation to the absence of alternatives they are very great. In about 5–10 per cent of cases the benefits are spectacular, e.g. the ability to recognise isolated words un-constrained by context (i.e. in open vocabulary sets), without lip-reading, and the ability to have a telephone conversation.

In comparison to the long-established services for which new developments are described in Chapters 3 and 4, cochlear implants are entirely 'new'. Clinical research done in the USA and Australia has given pointers sufficiently direct for specialised service units to be set up. In the UK during the 1980s, a handful of small cochlear implant programmes were set up as 'service developments' on charity funds. The Health Departments in England and Scotland established a 3-year centrally-funded service development programme in 1990, in nine centres including most of the existing charity-based ones anticipating a transition to regionally or supra-regionally funded services in 1993–4. Currently some dozen units in the UK provide a service—approximately double the number originally envisaged as being required.[7] Setting up a service was justified by international experience on a 'monitored implementation' basis rather than on a purely experimental basis. Evaluation of the service is fine-tuning the criteria for patient selection, and converging on cost-effective models for delivery. Given the existence of a service, important questions can now be answered about cochlear implantation, answers to which will shape the scale and nature of services in the future. Some types of public health question can only ethically be addressed once a service is in place. It is important to define the status of new services as neither purely experimental nor purely routine, but possessing elements of both; special funding arrangements may be needed to reflect this dual status. In return for earmarked funding, such units can reasonably be expected to co-operate with acquiring evaluation data at higher-than-typical levels of documentation, with the central transmission of data, and with working clinically to common protocols.

Clinical research on implantation has established a small number of major contraindications, including active middle-ear disease, an atrophied cochlea or cerebral cortex, or damage to the auditory nerve. After these exclusions have been made, the proportion of the remaining patients receiving no material benefit is now small enough that future research effort will concentrate on other questions. Absence of response to carefully executed non-implanted trial electrical stimulation is not currently taken as a contraindication, unless accompanying a cause suggesting no cochlear function such as head injury. This is because the test sensitivity has not been achieved that would justify declining the typical non-responder. However final stimulation can be useful in decisions on which ear to implant. The knowledge is not yet to hand to make valid decisions on whether or not to not implant a patient who is likely to receive **some** benefit but rather little. If it were possible to predict which patients receive only rather little benefit from a multi-channel intra-cochlear implant, then decisions could be better informed on the relative cost/benefit in each group of patients, and on the precise requirement in rehabilitation for each. Even with an accurate predication this would be invidious, although on the *triage* principle such decisions may eventually have to be made. The implications would depend on details of the individual case, but might involve investment in a cheaper single-channel implant, binaural acoustic hearing aids for those with useable hearing, or a vibrotactile aid, according to other predictive data. In fact such decisions between levels of technology are already being made, mainly on grounds of surgical feasibility. The mention of hearing aids here may seem surprising, if implants are supposed to be for those with no aidable hearing. This paradox leads to a poignant example of dilemma in distributive justice widely met in socialised medicine. Many people with enough hearing left to make some use of conventional acoustical aids tend (presumably because of the number of nerve fibres intact) to obtain great benefit from an implant, whereas those with only minimal or no auditory capacity tend to obtain modest benefit. Are treatment resources to be allocated according to absolute need or according to need measured as ability to benefit or some formula which reconciles the two? There is no easy answer to this question, although UK service development has tended to be geared primarily to absolute need.

Future possibilities

For the longer term the idea of individual prediction implies modifications of the general techniques of implantation and the associated rehabilitation to bring greater benefit to individual cases. For example, the currently favoured class of electrode design is geared to insertion through the round window at the base of the cochlea, which is coiled like a snail. Its manufacture accordingly involves an intrinsic degree of coiling matching that of the cochlea so as to facilitate insertion. However this technique permits insertion to only about two-thirds of the way up the coil, a limitation which entails inability to stimulate the low-frequency region of the cochlea directly. From the point of view of voice pitch (intonation) this does not matter greatly, because any frequency region can act as a carrier for the beating between voice harmonics that conveys low voice pitch. However, the arrangement is sub-optimal for the accurate coding of the full informative frequency spectrum of speech. The mapping of external frequency onto internal place of stimulation (and hence onto particular auditory nerve fibres) is constrained by maximum feasible insertion distance to involve a gap at low frequencies which in conventional psycho-acoustic terms leads to a hollow 'tinny' sound quality. One electrode mapping scheme involves re-introducing some of the missing low-frequency information by an upwards frequency shift, rather like playing a 33 RPM vinyl disc at 45 RPM. Implantees receiving this mapping make remarks at switch-on about a 'Donald Duck' quality to the speech they are hearing; this is one illustration of the challenge to learn to understand the slightly unnatural speech that the implant presents, one example of the need for rehabilitation. It is relatively easy to program variants in the external electronics of a general-purpose design for the speech-processing circuitry. The procedures for 'tuning up' individual patients already do this in simple ways, so as to guarantee most effective use of the inserted electrode contacts and some adequate mapping of the narrow dynamic range available between the threshold of audibility and the threshold of pain. Similar tailoring is not yet a reality for the hardware in the electrode array itself, but a tailoring effect is approximated in one implant system by providing a 22-channel electrode and selecting during the tune-up process a particular configuration of electrodes to stimulate. The options allowed by this redundancy tend to be used to achieve the maximum number of channels giving a response without discomfort rather than for sophisticated information mapping.

For surgical and physiological reasons, single-channel electrodes tend to be extra-cochlear whilst multi-channel ones tend to be intra-cochlear. This association is not absolutely essential and both types of counter-example exist. Techniques of drilling through bone from the outside onto multiple points on the inner ear went out of fashion in the early implant work for several reasons. However the possibility of accessing the nerve fibres in the hitherto unused apical (low-frequency) region of the inner ear may bring back such techniques, or some combination of conventional round-window insertion and drilling external to the cochlea in the temporal bone. This suggestion is made not for the sake of bio-engineering futurology, but for specific clinical reasons. Firstly, a more natural frequency mapping might reduce the initial re-learning period and hence reduce the requirement for rehabilitation; natural mapping will be helped by the inclusion of a low-frequency channel. Thus, subject to there being a sufficient minimum number of separately functioning channels, the external drilling approach should slightly raise performance for all implantees including the highest performers. Second, it could help those with poorest nerve fibre survival (and hence currently receiving rather little benefit from an implant), by maximising the range and hence the coverage of peripheral fibres, improving the resolution and dynamic range. Thirdly, inner ears which have filled with bony growth over the months and years since deafness began (especially when due to meningitis) are difficult to drill out in such a way as to enable the insertion of more than a few of the contacts on present-day multiple electrodes, and a rather limited benefit typically results. The external drilling approach might bring this group of patients up nearer to the average of present day levels of performance. (Where computed tomography reveals extensive bony growth within the cochlea, the current strategy for this group of patients is either to drill out the occupied spaces or to accept the more limited benefit from an extra-cochlear single-channel electrode; often however, the difficulty is only fully revealed at surgery.) Realisation of the potential of the external drilling approach depends critically upon whether electrodes can be brought close enough to nerve endings to keep down the necessary current levels and the current spread, and so avoid problems of narrow dynamic range and discomfort.

I have concentrated above on possible variants in electrode design and surgical approach, as these are linked to just over half of the total cost of providing an implant. In hearing, improvements in the service as a whole could follow from considering the requirements of subgroups of patients. There is, however, a difficulty—cost. The high investment costs for the manufacture of electrodes can only be recouped by using the methods of volume production and volume sale into a market that is in effect global. Production engineering to produce a variant on the electrode design would be almost as costly as for an entirely new type of electrode. Any special requirement of a group of patients that is smaller than about a third of the total market is thus unlikely to be met by commercial production, until technological progress has led to greatly reduced electrode production costs. The overall commercial viability of the entire cochlear implant industry is not yet so secure that specialised products could be carried at anything below the (very high) real costs of manufacture and distribution. At present, providers of health services are looking more to a reduction in the general price of electrodes than to sophisticated variations, and with the exception of the distinction intra-/extra-cochlear insertion, all existing implants are in direct competition. Indeed, current technological development work in the UK is directed primarily at lower-cost production of multi-channel implants having at least the performance of today's second generation. It is uncertain precisely where technological progress will be deployed in the future. The alternative paths are higher performance, cost reduction, greater flexibility, smaller size (for cosmetic reasons or to minimise invasiveness), and greater reliability, plus compliance with escalating standards and regulations.

New aspects of implant design will emerge to give higher benefit from third—than from second—generation devices: more numerous 'star' patients, and higher average performance throughout the range of performance achieved. The most notable scheme to emerge so far[8] separates the stimulation of the various electrode contacts in time as well as over place, so as to restrict mixing of currents between them. It works by interleaving (time-multiplexing), which requires a form of modulation onto a carrier periodicity higher than that to which auditory nerve fibres can respond directly. Such schemes can convey a more punctate, i.e. spectrally sharper, sensation and may slightly alleviate the problems of dynamic range.

Other trends in cochlear implant services can be anticipated as a result of current research and development. Firstly, results with young children, including children deaf from birth, look extremely promising in terms of accelerated development of communication skills.[9] There are good physiological reasons in the maturation of the nervous system why this should be so. Much has still to be learned about how best to use involuntary (objective) testing methods with young non-linguistic children, and how best to coax voluntary responses out of them. The objective assessments are necessary before implantation from a diagnostic point of view, but voluntary response techniques are also necessary to establish the baseline level of communication and language skills. For tuning the electrode map when habilitating the child and when monitoring progress, such techniques may also have some role, but only the voluntary response techniques are relevant. All these steps need to be undertaken in the most time-effective ways possible, but they require highly skilled specialised staff. It is regrettable that some implant programmes for children have been surgery-led rather than communication-led. However, some of the special problems with very young children **are** surgical and do demand definite extra skill (e.g. drilling in the shallow skull bone depth when accommodating the receiver package).

Service structures

Cochlear implant programmes are not currently highly integrated with rehabilitation services for profoundly deaf adults. The patients for such services include considerable numbers entering the referral process intended primarily for implants, but who turn out not to be suitable for an implant, or who decide eventually to decline surgery. Others arrive directly without any consideration of an implant. In an ideal world, cochlear implantation would have emerged as an appropriate constituent of a service providing comprehensive rehabilitation, rather than *vice versa*. However the world is not ideal, and it is now the task of audiologists and rehabilitation professionals to build upon and generalise the techniques found useful with implant patients, and to secure the continuation of more general rehabilitation services to adults and children and their wider provision to the group not suited to implants. This suggestion raises the problem of numbers, because the need for rehabilitation services is somewhat wider than that for implants. The much lower risks and costs of the non-implant devices required (high-power acoustical aids and vibrotactile aids) and the smaller number of specialising professionals required would justify a wider spread of local non-implanting rehabilitation units than of regional implanting units—perhaps two or three times the number. It is not clear how a sufficient number of rehabilitation units will come into existence without an initiative programme like that for implants, and there are only a handful in the UK currently acknowledged to have the relevant specialised experience and facilities.

The appropriate patient numbers (i.e. incidence of candidates meeting agreed criteria) in the UK cannot yet be given precise values. However, some lines of the argument about future provision are already very clear. Cochlear implantation does not come cheap. Detailed costings depend upon what overheads are included and on the amount of time spent in selection and rehabilitation; both of the latter bear directly on the quality of service, although there will be a point of diminishing returns all the sooner if the requirements are simple. Current estimates of benchmark real costs vary from £8,000 over and above the implant hardware cost for an 'easy' adult case, (giving a total around £20,000), up to over £30,000 in all (i.e. over £17,000 more than the hardware cost for a 'difficult' child). It would only be appropriate to begin comparing these figures with treatments in other areas where realistic (i.e. broad) overheads for general hospital facilities are included on both. It is not yet known what the maintenance or lifetime support costs are, and the issue of upgrades has not been addressed. For very young children it is not even clear yet where the 'initial provision' should be thought of as ending, and the 'subsequent lifetime' as beginning. This is a clinical research question, and also a financial one. It is to be hoped that the continuing costs turn out to be modest, and that effective ways can be found of accommodating the need for life-long support.

Amidst much uncertainty about costs and organisation, one course of events is highly predictable because it occurs so commonly. The realistic cost will understandably appear high to some purchasers. In the name of competition, the number of centres offering implantation will inevitably rise and cost-competition will lead to corner-cutting on selection and rehabilitation in the provider market. Some geographical spreading of services as they mature is generally justifiable, but this has to be constrained in proportion to the efficiency arising in concentrations of various forms of investment such as facilities and training. The concentration of rare skills (rather than the capital investment costs) must determine the level of aggregation at which services are organised. However in the extreme, cochlear implantation in every district general hospital would be manifestly absurd. Disagreement can enter on precisely where the lines should be drawn: about one implant centre per 5 million population, as the UK has now? About half this number, or twice this number? For partly laudible professional reasons, local providers wishing to offer a service themselves, particularly in the surgical aspects, will emphasise or may even exaggerate the financial advantage of spending the funds available closer to home (with the obviously genuine advantage of greater convenience to the patients) and now providers may even bid down charges with spurious claims of lower real costs. A poorer average service is likely to result from too much expansion, because of: (i) the inability to recruit adequately trained or sufficiently multidisciplinary staff, especially those involved in selection and rehabilitation, on which stages the corners will be cut; (ii) a lower caseload for each centre, which would be especially detrimental to the development and maintenance of the particular surgical skills; (iii) a shift of criteria for implantation more in the direction of including patients for implantation who would benefit from rehabilitation with less costly types of device; (iv) eventual financial non-viability of some centres and 'a market shakeout', which would in the event probably leave some patients needing to travel just as far for long-term support as if the local programme had not opened. This process would not necessarily remain efficient. Closure on grounds of non-profitability is the ultimate leveller and stabiliser in truly competitive markets, but in health, such market oscillations could be expected to occur only rather slowly. The imperfect market envisaged for the Health Service as yet has little provision for circulating information about levels of the quality of 'products' nor of the professional experience and skill that supposedly underlie quality. It might leave inefficient and/or low-quality services in place for several years, without necessarily guaranteeing survival of the most cost-effective.

Some slight expansion in the number of cochlear implant centres beyond the dozen or so currently serving the UK could be clinically effective and efficient in the use of skilled staff resources, if it occurred in conjunction with more widespread provision for non-implant selection and rehabilitation, which is already needed. It is likely that the 'provider push' will continue to come primarily from individual surgeons wishing to do the surgery, somewhat irrespective of the rehabilitative and economic context. The surgical caseload and the skills exercised upon it would need to be considered carefully and concentrated, e.g. a combined team of four surgeons from two linked hospitals, rather than two from one. Nevertheless, from the point of view of cost, quality, safety and effectiveness, it will be necessary to avoid a proliferation of implant centres. It is problematic how far (in the long-term) the number of UK centres should rise beyond the current dozen or so, unless it is found that demand (from appropriate candidates) markedly exceeds capacity, or unless cochlear implant centres are rolled into a wider rehabilitation initiative.

Post-implementation research

The frequency discussion illustrates the complexity of the issues faced in research and development that impact upon issues of policy, planning and public health. Usually clinical research alone is insufficient to address them and post-implementation evaluative research is required. To give an impression of the diversity of issues in post-implementation research in cochlear implants, Table 5.1 lists six questions about cochlear implant services that require to be answered. This list is far from exhaustive; in particular it does not include any of the bioengineering and clinical research questions that are currently driving the development of third-generation hardware. The table also makes a general point about the sorts of specific reason for which post-implementation research is required.

The Health Departments for England and Scotland have commissioned from the MRC Institute of Hearing Research an evaluation of the centrally funded cochlear implant programme in the nine centrally funded centres. Among the questions that the evaluation will answer are those in the table. The data to be gathered embrace the medical and psychological background to selection, cost and process data on the services provided, a wide range of performance tests to measure the benefits of electro-auditory stimulation upon communication, and a range of questionnaire measures of communication and quality of life. The evaluation study can not point to a precise ideal number of implanting centres, but should indicate a sensible range to aim at, subject to the unfolding of further considerations in the light of economic and technological progress. At the time of writing, data from the evaluation are not yet available, but some observations can be made about the role of such evaluations that may be of longer-lived importance than the results of a particular evaluation study.

Evaluation can take many forms, so the term has no single fixed meaning. Evaluation is relatively new to health services in the UK, and especially new in the form where it is built into the fabric

TABLE 5.1 *Questions for post-implementation research—cochlear implants*

1. How great and how diverse are the benefits of cochlear implants in adults?*⁎
2. Which types of patient benefit most? + ⁎
3. What are the fixed and the variable costs?†@*
4. At what rate do suitable patients come forward; hence what are the backlog and the projected service incidence?* + @
5. Does the contrast in a pragmatic trial between extended (or intensive) and slight rehabilitation suggest that the former is more (cost-) effective. And is a further, controlled, trial required? + @⁎
6. What are the risks and complications of implantation* + @†⁎

The reasons why post-implementation research is required to supplement basic demonstrations of benefit in clinical research distribute over the main objective of the UK cochlear implant programme as follows:

* Realistic (service) circumstances of implantation.

\+ Large numbers of patients—not highly selected.

@ Multi-centre study.

† Long-term follow-up.

⁎ More clinical documentation than routine service, with appropriate outcome measures.

of a programme from the start. In much of continental Europe clinical research, evaluation and audit are at such a rudimentary level that it is even unclear how the literature in English can best be translated. In this respect the USA is far ahead, and its attitude to experimental programmes with evaluation has always been more scientific than the traditional UK one of delaying implementation till political groundswell or the weight of loosely gathered experience push towards universal implementation. Evaluations can include some elements of three more familiar processes—the formal clinical trial, the informal appraisal of a new programme that will require significant investment by centres beyond those of its origin, and the assessment of specific pieces of new health technology by third parties who are neither buying nor selling it.

Evaluations built into the initial planning of programmes seem to offer five distinct advantages: (i) The appropriate form of the evaluation is thought out and planned at the outset, not as an afterthought. (ii) A set of decision points is scheduled, along with a general indication or agreement on the way in which subsequent decisions will use the data to be gathered. (iii) Objectives and processes are clarified and specified at the start (as in clinical trials), leading to greater efficiency, consensus and standardisation in the programme itself. (iv) The tools of the evaluation, e.g. tests, proformas, and clinical database, become tools of the programme also. (v) The data provide a baseline and framework for subsequent clinical audit on a continuing and widespread basis, as well as providing answers to the major strategic questions at the end of the programme. This assists the accommodation of practical experience in the particular area of innovation. Points (iii) and (iv) should be beneficial to the quality of programmes evaluated in 'built-in' fashion, although they build a new type of uncertainty principle into the entire enterprise of evaluation. Hence generalisation about the quality of programme that can be obtained after the evaluation phase is complete may have to be cautious. Point (v) may assist here by enabling the issue to be addressed over a wider site of providers and over the longer term.

Returning to the specific instance of cochlear implants, it is virtually certain that the next decade will see higher levels of communication performance being achieved by some users of cochlear implants. Beyond that, forecasting is difficult. Whether clinical criteria for candidature become broadened in relation to benefits from rehabilitative regimes based on acoustical and vibro-tactile aids will depend upon costs and on the interplay of finance and organisation discussed earlier: in a cash-limit rationing system expensive treatments may have to be reserved for those for whom there are **no** real alternatives. Because of the importance of the prevalence/severity distribution, any broadening of criteria will lead to a large increase in the numbers of candidates on an incidence basis. The balance of demonstrated advantage for hearing losses in the range 90–105 dB HL is shifting fairly firmly towards implantation. More depends on the financial climate.

This section has attempted to describe the complex set of considerations involved in setting up a new service for a high-cost high-technology treatment and in anticipating how it can and should evolve. There is nothing new or unique to cochlear implants in this, but the arrival of these big-league issues in audiology/ENT has been startling, and the lack of precedent may make the professional response idiosyncratic. Over the decades, dissemination and expectations have increased, and the fruits of discoveries are wanted in the local hospital the week after they first appear in the general news media. Therefore an overall under-standing of the interrelationship of the technological, clinical, epidemiological and financial/organisation issues is necessary to forecast and steer developments.

Formal posing of research questions has an important role in deciding issues in each of these spheres, even those of finance and organisation, but it is difficult to frame all aspects of the issues in testable hypotheses and often expensive then to test them. A framework of rationale must therefore relate the issues, and that is what I have attempted to give. It is better that such a rationale be concerned to link maximally to research findings and known principles, than that it should emerge exclusively from interested parties, such as service providers, as was the case in the past.

3. HEALTH SERVICES RESEARCH

For the mainstream of hearing services described in Chapters 3 and 4 it is hard to envisage innovations in the next decade as radical in form as those just discussed. Most types of innovation need to be translated into an improvement in the corresponding service by performing the respectively appropriate type of health services research (HSR). HSR addresses issues of need, benefit (effectiveness), supply, demand, cost, efficiency, acceptability, quality and optimum mode of delivery in health care.[10] Such issues have been close to the surface both in Chapter 3 (cost/effectiveness in the early detection of hearing disorders in children) and in Chapter 4 (prevalence of need for auditory rehabilitation, demand, and supply). The discussion of future de-velopments in hereditary deafness and cochlear implants has emphasised the interrelations of basic biomedical research and development with the HSR stages—i.e. with evaluation, or other types of post-implementation research. Thus in all my chosen topic areas, HSR issues have permeated the biomedical and clin-ical research agendas and *vice versa*. As an example of the need for HSR, developments can enter practice on the basis of fashion, only to generate widespread waste and eventual rejection. Rejec-tion of a technique or element of service usually occurs on grounds of redundancy (especially in diagnostic techniques), of insufficient cost-effectiveness or time-effectiveness, or of poor investment timing in relation to the arrival of better techniques. Leaving aside examples of quackery and treatments without rationale, rarely is a **total** absence of any utility or benefit the reason for rejection. Accepting this implies an acceptance that mere demonstration of **some** utility is far from a justification for the adoption of a new procedure or piece of technology; the magnitude of the effect must be documented on some scale with known benchmarks. This last observation is a powerful argument that research should increasingly assess magnitude of benefits in relation to service costs. Unfortunately, this is yet one more pressure making research itself more costly, because a study to estimate magnitude accurately has to be several times larger than one merely demonstrating the existence of some effect in a particular direction. The lore of nicely calculated 'less' or 'more', may be rejected in Heaven (according to William Wordsworth) but it is a grinding necessity here on Earth.

Systematic HSR is vital if appropriate services are to exist, evolve, and play an appropriate part in the quality of life and the national economy. HSR embraces many different types of research: the epidemiology of need, the later generalisation and optimisation stages of clinical trials, health technology assessment, the systemisation and evaluation of professional skills, operational studies of the efficient structuring and flow of work and of patients through health care systems, the economics of heatlh care, and the behavioural factors in maintaining individuals' health including their uptake of services. Even this diverse list is not exhaustive and these areas in turn draw upon rather diverse types of academic discipline. HSR supplements clinical research, leading to established principles whereby one 'good-practice' model can be preferred over another.

Composing the HSR agenda

The way in which services evolved and expanded in the past was largely provider-led, and had some arbitrary elements. The ageing population, a greater awareness and expectation, and the increasing potential from expensive medical technologies have made growth in demand outstrip the growth in resources and the supply of services. The allocation of paramount status to questions of effectiveness and the prioritisation of services to be provided is very recent. The inevitable excess of demand over supply makes an analytic approach to services as a whole essential for resource allocation, the related manpower planning, and the evolution of professional roles and training. Whatever role market forces may be allocated in the mechanisms of supply, these issues will need to be faced in setting the scale of demand that can be met. However, the quantity of detailed suitable information that has been acquired for use in decision-making for effectiveness remains regrettably small. Although already increasing as a result of Health Department initiatives, the quantity of HSR in the UK remains modest as a percentage of the NHS budget. The quantity of such research in hearing disorders has been particularly small, although one UK tradition interested in the process of auditory rehabilitation has been interested also in some issues of service delivery—the rough costs, the coverage and effectiveness of services—in addition to issues of clinical procedure.

The ideal generator process for HSR is a sequence of study stages, rather than a single prototypical design or style of study. A new service ingredient or package is: (i) proposed on the basis of new or existing knowledge, often derived from basic biomedical work; (ii) optimised by a variety of small-scale, sometimes informal, studies to a level where it can be specified as contrasting with specifiable alternatives; and then (iii) subjected to controlled trial, pragmatic trial or observational evaluation to see whether the innovation is better than the prevailing standard arrangements (or better than none at all). Let us consider what could be meant by 'better'—some combination of: more beneficial, more precisely selective of those in need, more deliverable, more sparing of skilled labour (or in other ways less costly), more efficient (including the reduction of other displaced costs), more free of side-effects, or more productive of feelings of satisfaction. The particularly appropriate combination of all these indicators has to be determined by the context. For example, in a professional category where recruiting and retaining staff is already a prime problem, modifications to procedures or new equipment have to be given priority—modifications that may de-skill* a procedure or

*The choice of de-skilling as an example may appear politically loaded to some readers but is not. Whether for reasons of training, recruitment or salary costs, skills at high level will always be in short supply; the point is to deploy them where they are most needed (as noted in Chapter 4). It is necessary also, when proposing a new service, to properly assess the skill requirement with its impact upon quality, and hence not to underestimate the costs (as noted in Chapter 3).

permit it to be substituted by another deliverable by a different professional group, while maintaining or increasing the overall health gain in relation to the total resources committed. In research and development on the activities of a professional group in short supply, these considerations might sometimes take precedence as outcome measures over issues of benefit, or over reduction in other forms of cost. In this way the science in HSR has to be both opportunistic as to feasibility and pragmatic as to need. Although engineers and inventors never suffered from reluctance to welcome these constraints onto their agenda, the practitioners of basic science have often thought development issues to be unworthy of their inattention, and have been less willing to regard socio-technical systems as a worthy topic for analytic skills.

Pursuing the agenda

Under most circumstances the rigorous demonstration of effectiveness is surprisingly complicated, for a long list of methodological reasons that there is space only to hint at. In evaluations and clinical trials, four related effects can combine to reduce the apparent size of treatment effect demonstrable, by raising the obtained average on the outcome measures for the baseline condition (i.e. for the individuals or the service units that serve as control). These four artefactual effects are: (i) the 'Hawthorne' effect, whereby personnel under observation work with more motivation, e.g. actually or fully following all the already recommended procedures; (ii) the placebo effect, whereby patients given careful attention and explanation, and an expectation of benefit, will experience subjective benefit or psychosomatic alleviation, even when no 'treatment' with a possibly effective ingredient has been included; (iii) the contamination or ripple effect, which occurs mostly when the treatments compared are based in knowledge, procedure and information, rather than in some wholly controllable pill or operation; here the knowledge that contributes to the procedure under test may 'escape' from the index patients, units or districts and migrate along professional networks to the control ones, because the procedure is plausibly a good new idea; and (iv) the trials effect, whereby even patients from whom the new treatment is withheld in clinical trials appear to fare better than background non-trial patients do.[11] The trials effect may not always be genuine, but where it is that probably arises in part from a Hawthorne effect (higher general standard of care). There are other possible explanations, such as uncontrolled selection of patients and careful selection of collaborators in trials. As discussed above, circumstances may require a combination of controlled designs with observational design to overcome these difficulties. It is ironic that the four artefactual effects are a great threat to conclusive and generalisable research, but are important vehicles of effective medicine and of effective management in organisations.

The intellectual and practical resources required for demonstrating what works best are great; such research can be more difficult to do than laboratory research, and doing it well is costly. But the personnel resources for doing evaluations and HSR generally are in short supply.[12] As a consequence, the demand for trials or evaluation of service packages or ingredients has to be kept in proportion. That demand can be attenuated under four circumstances: (i) where the regime is of low risk, non-contentious, rational and of low cost per individual; (ii) where it is dramatically effective, whilst of low risk; (iii) where the total resources involved, given a low incidence of the condition in question, are modest; and (iv) where there is an ethical imperative to do something for the patient, the treatment is of low risk, and no effective alternatives can be envisaged. Any of these four combinations of circumstance can allow a particular form of provision to go ahead while placing it at the back of the queue for evaluation resources or attenuating the rigour and cost of the evaluation imposed. As a coarse dichotomy for handling this distinction, I distinguish minimal but acceptable palliative care (MAPC) from specific cost-effective treatments (SCET). The term 'minimal' simply describes the typical resource level and is not intended to imply that level of care should be forced down to the minimum that will be accepted at a particular place and time. Clearly the evaluation requirement differs radically between MAPC and SCET.

Motivation for HSR Studies

The development of most health services for the hearing-impaired in the near future should involve a three-part process: (a) gradual small-scale improvement of ingredients such as fitting procedures for hearing aids through biomedical research and technological development; (b) combining of these elements into proposed packages and refinement of the candidature criteria for individuals' receipt of these; and (c) comparative trials of packages or major elements in packages to document cost and benefit (limited according to the four principles of attenuation above). This scenario is hardly novel, but working through a hypothetical example shows a major problem in doing the style of research now required. As a thought-experiment, let us consider the following sketch of a study on hearing aids to evaluate the proposal that some specific candidate group might fare better than they would with a standard instrument, if they were to be provided with a hearing aid having an extended high-frequency response and smoothly varying amplifier gain across frequency—in other words, a hi-fi aid. Before taking in the example design, the reader may wish to look back over the section in Chapter 4 on hearing aids. Specific candidates for the hi-fi aid and a group of non-specific candidates would be identified differing in audiometric characteristics; otherwise they would have similar characteristics. Non-specific candidates, i.e. the wider group of candidates for a standard aid would be included, partly as control against placebo, partly against a non-specific 'better-overall' effect for the more sophisticated aid, and partly to clarify cost implications if a 'better-overall' effect were indeed to be found. The amount of counselling advice towards toleration of the initially harsher and less pleasant sounds from the extended-frequency aid might be included as an extra variable, at least for those receiving the extended frequency-response. Measures of initial use-time, plus the user's volume-and tone-control settings, would be taken to throw light on the effect of this counselling. In principle, such an investigation should include appropriate multiple outcome measures to provide a pooled measure of benefit and hence to be able to define points on a cost-benefit function. This would enable a judgement about the extra benefit, for the specific candidate group, from the extended-frequency aid in relation to the extra cost. As a preparation for decisions, this marginal cost-benefit might be interpreted against wider norms of cost-benefit (for example with standard provision to both groups) and compared with other proposals for how marginal benefits could be increased.

On the face of it, I have given a purely technical (i.e. audiological) description of a plausible study. However it illustrates a profound dilemma in the planning and **motivation** of HSR studies. Each new element of health services is inevitably, if indirectly, competing with other new elements and some existing ones. In such a world studies like the one outlined are essential to wise health investment. It is important to note that they have not often been done, and to realise why not. A main reason lies in the requirement for combined sophistication in matters of hearing aid technology, in measurements of performance and satisfaction, and in health economics. Ironically, one further reason is similar to the prototypical circumstances that **necessitate** clinical trials, and which can help to justify them and secure the ethical agreement to withhold treatment in controls—i.e. a well-documented division of opinion on the issue. However in this instance, the potential division is not the usual type of disagreement where one school of providers and another come together to agree on what data could resolve their disagreement; rather it is between two different classes of player—the purchasers and providers of services. The division also concerns not the **direction** of the evidence, but the need for the study and the magnitude of effect sought. Many audiologists, i.e. providers, would regard the main idea behind the study sketched above, for differential prescription of hearing aids, as already accepted, subject perhaps to some fine-tuning of precisely who should be considered a candidate. Providers might thus think the value of a study of the type suggested was low, even if it were to be well executed; they might regard it as redundant upon clinical experience or repetitive of scattered results from small studies that already allow a reasonably accurate prediction that the technologically 'better' aid is indeed better in its outcomes for the specific candidate group. This misapprehension is particularly encouraged by mentally storing the results of past in a verbal form work as sentences—propositions thought to be true—from abstracts drawing qualitative conclusions. On the other hand, the accessibility, amount, certainty, pervasiveness, scaling and quantitative precision of such research done to date, plus its lack of a public health perspective, probably falls short of what would convince a procurement executive to contract for a special class of hearing aid or convince a director of public health and his or her advisers to fund an enlarged service. The result of these differing perspectives is an *impasse*. The topic may not be seen as novel enough to attract those whose primary function is research; (for this reason any article reporting such a study might require a clearly stated and even over-critical emphasis on the limitations of interpretation of previous evidence, in order to justify the study and hence to secure publication on novelty grounds). Some providers who are active only part-time in research might not be too concerned about this issue of novelty, but this group might equally lack the perspective or inclination to formulate a new project in the health-economic way required by the purchaser.

Need for an 'Evaluation Culture'

Ineffective or inefficient elements of services can survive due to wishful thinking, stereotypes, or inertia, and due to providers' or suppliers' vested interests going unexamined. Such errors of **commission** are common throughout health services. They show up particularly in variations in medical practice, which are a major source of inefficiency, even if they do not always have direct consequences in variation in health gain. In a particular field at a particular time the difficult strategic judgement may need to be made whether the difficulties in formal trials of effectiveness of specified procedures should be faced, or whether the study of and eventual compression of practice variations[13] by practice guidelines and audit may be more appropriate to the problem. As pointers to the continuing need for research in the area of the disabilities, we must anticipate that errors of **omission** will accumulate in the years to come. Services for disabled people including the hearing-impaired will not be upgraded and can be expected specifically to suffer from difficulties of access to the scarce motivation, skills and resources in research that is now required if the effectiveness of rational proposals for new elements of services are to be documented as effective. Nevertheless, following Pascal's wager, there is little alternative to optimistic belief that an adequate amount of evaluative research will somehow be done. Services built up painstakingly over many years will not necessarily be pared away immediately, even if they seem vulnerable on the grounds that the era in which they and their related training were built up did not demand, or offer facilities for, research on outcomes and health gain.

For the majority of paediatric and adult audiology in the 1990s, i.e. broadly the areas described in Chapters 3 and 4, performing the appropriate HSR could be as great an engine of progress as radical innovation. However, there are other forces for change than the formation of effective service models based on results of biomedical and clinical research. Pure technological push, or changes arising from economic or personnel factors, will continue to drive many changes. Indeed, the instigation of HSR rarely comes out of an individual's opportunistic search for contexts in which to do the more elegantly controlled among HSR projects. Rather, there is a pooled awareness of a major need for information on costs, effectiveness, risks or other uncertainties of new technology; these, balanced with some parochial opportunities and priorities, eventually push particular HSR projects to the top of individuals' or organisations' agendas.

Scientific opportunism will be vital in HSR as in basic research, in two respects. Opportunities for the fruitful comparison of index patients and systems (i.e. those that are receiving the treatment under evaluation) with controls (i.e. the standard, baseline, untreated) have to be discerned or created. Such opportunities arise for example where two hospitals or districts have similar populations, facilities, staffing and professional content of the service, but the additional ingredient under scrutiny can be provided in one not the other; these favourable circumstances are few and have to be carefully cultivated. Unfortunately, distance between sites in a trial or evaluation study, although it assists the control of variables through reducing contamination, increases the administrative overheads and makes it less likely that a single regional health authority can adopt and execute many research plans of the scale required. A second important instance of opportunism involves the appreciation of the narrow time window for evaluation of new developments (with expensive technologies in particular). Here the development has to have become sufficiently interesting to the relevant profession to be worth evaluating, in order to generate co-operation and some resource input from the co-operation of the early practitioners; it is possible to start too soon as well as too late. Whether benefits are substantial or not, the window passes once the development has become so widespread as to be regarded as having virtually entered conventional practice; even if the research remains feasible and ethical, its results may arrive too late to influence events.

The potential cumulative benefits and cost savings in an enterprise of the scale of the UK National Health Service justify investments in research into major questions, on a scale much larger than has been seen in the past. The new arrangements for research and development in the Health Service which began in 1991 stem from this realisation, and will play an increasing role in tackling the immense challenges of costs, organisation, quality and effectiveness presented to the Health Service in the 1990s. Despite a good tradition of concern with issues of need and cost in British audiology, research that seeks to underpin, or which optimises services for hearing-impaired people, currently shows signs of missing this evolution through isolation from the mainstream of public health issues. An opportunity may be missed, to the detriment of services for hearing-impaired people. I hope that this monograph serves to diminish that isolation.

REFERENCES

1. FRASER, G., (1976). *The causes of profound deafness in childhood.* London, Baillière Tindall.
2. STEEL, K. P., (1991). 'Similarities between mice and humans with hereditary deafness'. In RUBEN, J. R., VAN DE WATER, T. R., AND STEEL, K. P., (Eds). 'Genetics of Hearing Impairment'. *Annals of the New York Academy of Sciences,* **630**, 68–79.
3. JORDAN, I. K., (1991). 'Ethical issues in the genetic study of deafness'. In RUBEN, J. R., VAN DE WATER, T. R., AND STEEL, K. P., (Eds). 'Genetics of Hearing Impairment'. *Annals of the New York Academy of Sciences,* **630**, 236–239.
4. SHAVER-ARNOS, K., ISRAEL, J., AND CUNNINGHAM, D. R., (1991). 'Ethical issues on the genetic study of deafness'. In RUBEN, J. R., VAN DE WATER, T. R., AND STEEL, K. P., (Eds). 'Genetics of Hearing Impairment'. *Annals of the New York Academy of Sciences,* **630**, 317–318.
5. TYLER, R. S., (1990). 'The performance of post-lingually deafened adults with cochlear implants. In HAGGARD, M. P., AND PAGE, M., (Eds). 'Clinical Developments in Cochlear Implants. Southampton'. *Duphar Medical,* (ISBN-1-870678-25-7).
6. BILGER, R. C., (1977). 'Psycho-acoustic evaluation of present prostheses'. *Annals of Otology, Rhinology and Laryngology,* **86** (Suppl 38), 92–140.

7. THORNTON, A. R. D., (1986). 'Estimation of the number of patients who might be suitable for cochlear implant and similar procedures'. *British Journal of Audiology*, **20**, 221–229.
8. STALLER, S. J., BEITER, M., BRIMACOMBE, J. H., MECKLENBURG, D. J., AND ARNDT, P., (1991). 'Paediatric performance with the Nucleus 22-channel cochlear implant system'. *American Journal of Otology*, 12 (Suppl), 126–136.
9. WILSON, B. S., FINLEY, C., LAWSON, D. J., WOLFORD, R. D., EDDINGTON, D. K., AND RASINOUTZ, W. M., (1991). 'Better speech recognition with cochlear implants'. *Nature*, **352**, 236–238.
10. MECHANIC, D., (1978). 'Prospects and problems in Health Services Research'. *Millbank Quarterly/Health and Society*, **56**(2).
11. KARJALAINEN, S., AND PALVA, I., (1989). 'Do treatment protocols improve end results? A study of survival of patients with multiple myeloma in Finland'. *British Medical Journal*, **299**, 1069–72.
12. CLARKE, M., AND KURINCZUK, J. J., (1992). 'Health Services Research: a case of need or special pleading? *British Medical Journal*, **304**, 1675–1676.
13. ANDERSEN, T. F., AND MOONEY, G., (Eds). (1990). *The challenge of Medical Practice Variations*. London, Macmillan.